The Beginner Vegan Athlete

Carol Capper

Carol Capper

ISBN: 9798391681182

Carol Capper

Living a vegan lifestyle has many different benefits. Backed up by multiple prominent research studies, it has been proven that a vegan lifestyle can lower the risk of cardiac events, reduce the risk of developing certain cancers and lower an individual's chance of type 2 diabetes. It also helps regulate one's metabolism and weight and stave off certain weight-induced phenomena, such as hypertension. A vegan lifestyle has also been proven to reduce someone's risk of stroke.

Why   Go   Vegan?

But, there are many benefits to a vegan lifestyle that are not merely based on health. The UN recently released a report that stated a dire need for the world to migrate away from consistently consuming animal products. The impact of most of the growing population consuming meat and animal products is the growing need for crops to feed those animals and breed them for food.

Food is not like finding an alternative to fossil fuels. People are required to eat for their survival. However, as the current population stands, animals raised to provide food to the general population consume over half of the world's crops.

Yes, half.

And no, that is not some random statistic. That statistic was embedded within the UN's official report.

It is simply an inefficient use of our planet's natural resources. As the population continues to grow because of advancements in medicine, more agricultural space will be necessary to grow and feed the heightened number of animals bred for food purposes. Many people talk about deforestation and scream for it to go away. Still, many people do not understand that around 56% of that deforestation is going to the purpose of agriculture: growing food not simply for humans but for those animals that are raised specifically for general food sources.

And, as if that is not enough, around 850,000,000 people (around 15% of the world's population) struggle and deal with undernourishment, even with all of this. If we continue, it is simply a waste of the planet's natural resources that will become exhausted soon.

What does being vegan have to do with any of this? Not consuming animal products and meat take a bit of the burden off this need for more agricultural space for those animals we need to feed. Adopting a vegan lifestyle takes the stress off the planet's natural resources and will ultimately require less water, fossil fuels, and land to cultivate.

DEDICATION

This book is dedicated to the one who started me on the vegan journey
decades ago. Thank You!

Carol Capper

Disclaimer Notice:

Please note that the information contained within this document is for educational and entertainment purposes only. Every attempt has been made to provide accurate, up-to-date, reliable, and complete information. No warranties of any kind are expressed or implied. Readers acknowledge that the author does not render legal, financial, medical, or professional advice.

By reading this document, the reader agrees that under no circumstances are we responsible for any direct or indirect losses incurred due to the use of the information contained within this document, including, but not limited to, errors, omissions, or inaccuracies.

Table of Contents

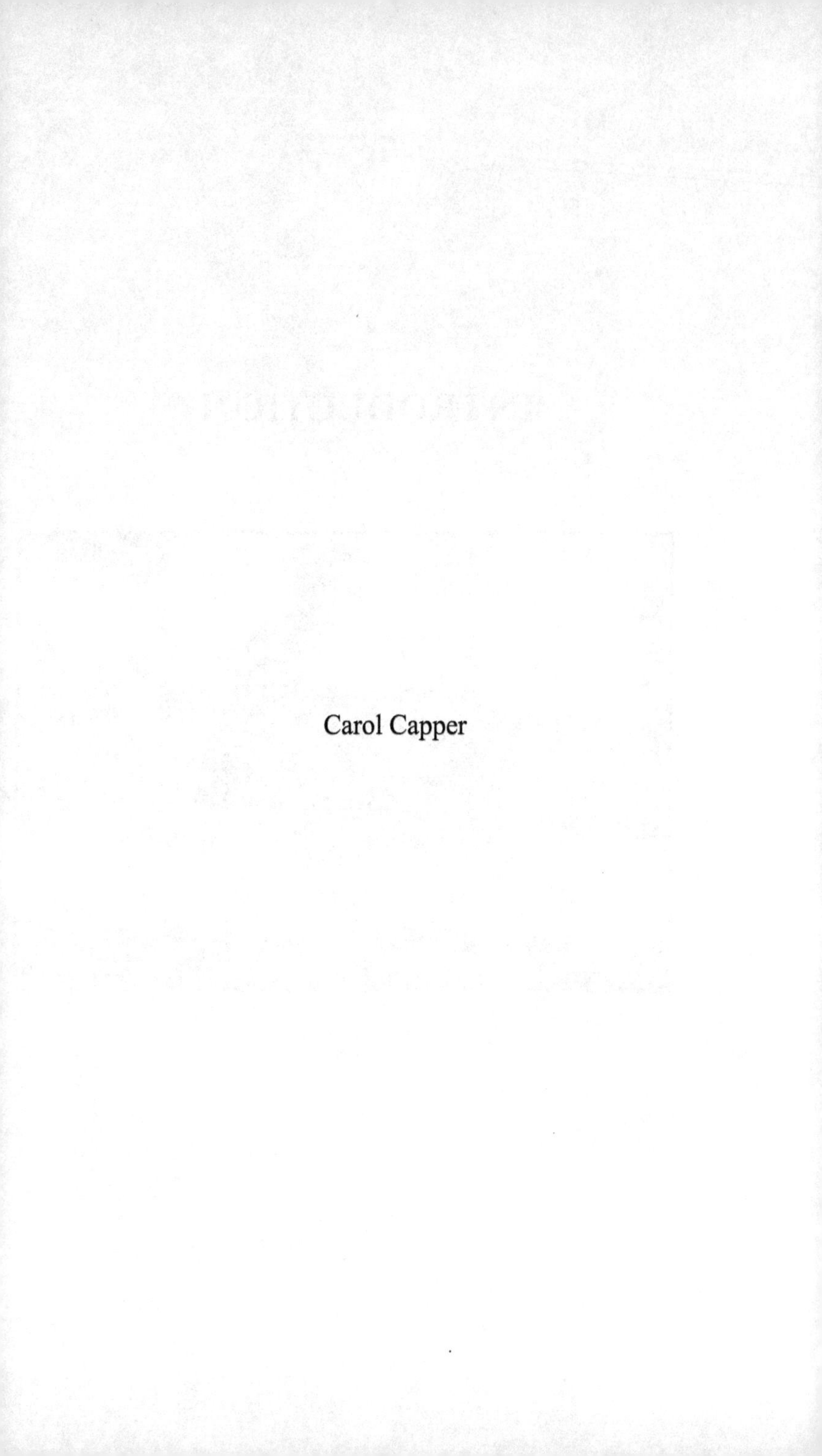

Carol Capper

INTRODUCTION

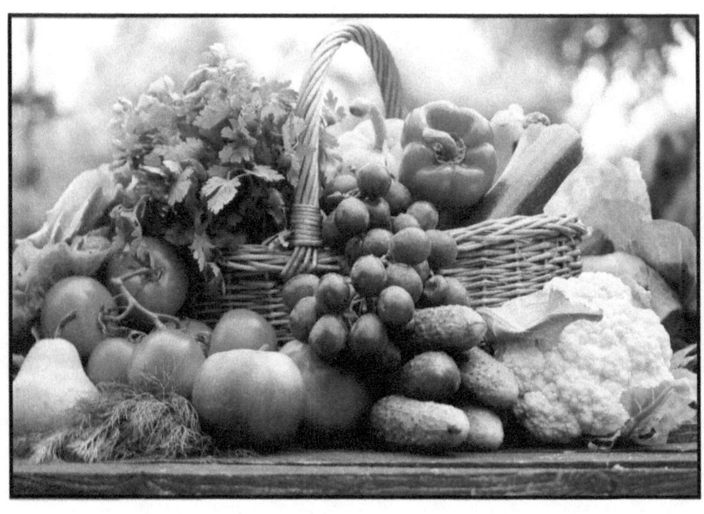

> *"The Vegan Athlete: Athletic Outline"* contains proven steps
> and strategies on how to begin your vegan diet, how to
> maintain and acquire the type of body you wish on a vegan
> diet, and presents to you athletes and prominent individuals
> who debunk some of the greatest myths when it comes to the
> world of vegan eating.

Many believe a vegan lifestyle is not conducive to muscle building or psychological health.

Many believe vegans cannot possibly obtain the protein sources they need to keep their bodies working efficiently, and others believe that a vegan lifestyle should not be held for the long haul. Many people are under the assumption that to live a healthy and productive life inside (and outside) of the gym; one has to chug protein shakes and energy supplements to improve performance consistently.

We are here to let you know that none of these are true. This book will have real-life athletes who not only live a vegan lifestyle but prove that performance and muscle-building are not simply based on the idea of laboratory-manufactured and animal-based protein sources. This book will talk about the true dietary needs of vegans and where they get their sources from. It will compare the types of nutrients and proteins other dietary lifestyles obtain to show that vegans do not simply go without; they choose to broaden their food-based horizon.

Not only that, but many believe that a vegan lifestyle cannot give someone the energy they need to work out in a gym for two hours. Well, not only will this be another myth debunked within the pages of this book, but it will also be something we address in full. That is, we will outline various workout plans and routines that will benefit the vegan lifestyle you have chosen (or are, at least, curious about) to achieve the physical benefits you want for your own body.

Yes, it is possible to build muscle on a vegan diet, and it is possible to keep up those cardio-based marathons on a vegan diet. You will be genuinely surprised at how similar the workout routine is for those who "eat vegan" and those who do not.

Vegans are not individuals who shove their beliefs down someone's throat. They are individuals who are merely passionate about abstaining from using animal products. They do not consume them; some individuals even attempt not to use them. Are there extremists? Yes, but there are extremists in every healthy lifestyle.

Within the pages of this book will be dietary outlines for those who are (or want to be) vegan, exercise guidelines for those eating this type of food lifestyle, and athletes that will be real-life examples of how this works. Not only that, but these athletes will have their testimonies as to why they began this lifestyle and how it has benefitted them in the long run.

And, as if that was not enough, all of those dreaded myths perpetuated about the vegan lifestyle will finally be debunked.

Welcome to the new and amazing world of vegan fitness and nutrition.

CHAPTER 1

A VEGAN VOYAGE FOR WELL-BEING AND PERFORMANCE

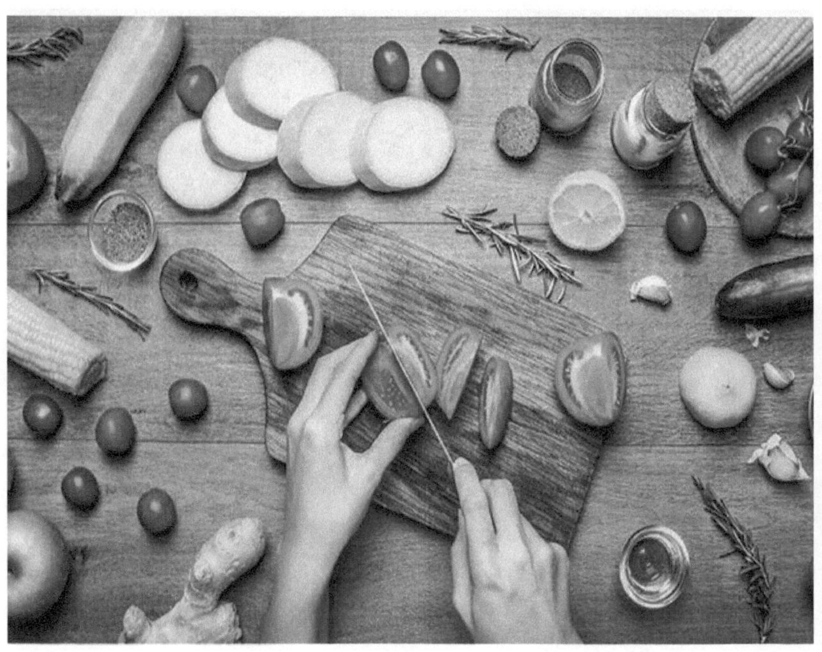

Multiple reports have surfaced that declare the world's population will be around 9 billion individuals by 2050. Many more studies have been done that proclaim the world's meat needs will not be sustainable by that point.

Adopting a vegan lifestyle can help that statistic.

The Immense Benefits

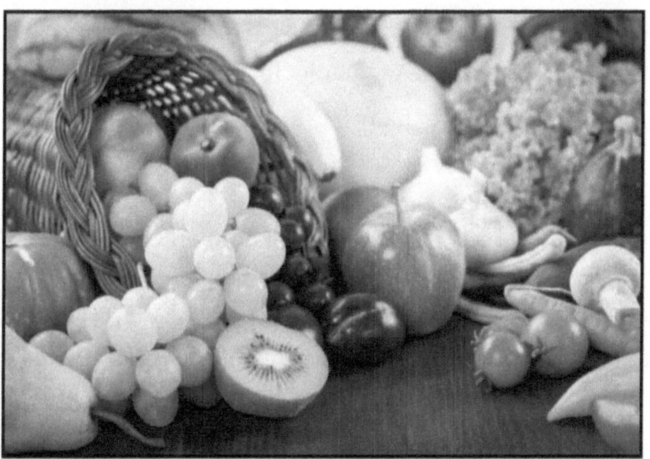

Many vegans scream about animal cruelty and how that should be the reason everyone converts to a vegan lifestyle. Still, the truth is that more people are concerned about their well-being rather than the well-being of an animal they cannot see, touch or hear. So, it should bring a smile to many people's faces when we say there are more scientifically-backed studies that give even more personal health benefits that are only provided when adopting a vegan diet.

It has been shown in various studies that a vegan diet provides higher availability of fiber, potassium, antioxidants, and folate, which makes it the most mineral-

and-vitamin-rich diet offered on the health and wellness circuit today. Not only that, but it is the number one recommended diet by general physicians and specialists when it comes to someone who needs to lose weight. One particularly renowned study compared a vegan diet to a dozen other popular and well-received diets and found that the participants who adopted the vegan diet lost the most weight, with an average of 9.3 pounds more than all the other groups of participants utilizing other diets!

It can also help level out blood sugar levels and promote kidney function by lowering and regulating internal blood sugars. It has been proven to help individuals who suffer from different arthritic pains because many vegetables and fruits ingested contain antioxidants and free radicals (yes, those are a thing) that help manage internal swelling.

However, no one can deny the social stigma and misconceptions many people have because of the loud-and-proud vegans who accuse people of being monsters because they eat meat. Unfortunately, they are out there. With any lifestyle, whether health-based, politically-based, or religiously-based, comes those who take it to an extreme and give the lifestyle a bad reputation. Luckily, there are ways you can combat that social stigma should you choose to adopt a vegan diet and/or lifestyle.

Do Your Research – Seek The Truth

For starters, educate yourself. Look into those studies and hold those statistics at the ready. With taboo subjects come people who want you to "prove" what you are discussing. So, be ready. Read and educate yourself in the avenues that have proven a vegan lifestyle does what it claims to do.

Many other people believe vegans are not getting what they need regarding macro-and-micro nutrients. Take, for example, protein and calcium. Once someone hears someone does not eat meat or animal byproducts, they automatically assume two things are not being ingested: calcium from milk and protein from meat. This is another avenue to educate someone properly.

Use your thirst for knowledge and research foods rich in calcium and protein that are not stereotypical resources. Not only should you incorporate those into your diet, but you can also use this information when educating someone on veganism versus what they were originally introduced to.

Another way to get around this social stigma if you have not fully educated yourself is to say you enjoy the taste of something while not enjoying the taste of something else. If you go out to a restaurant and order a vegan-based dish, someone will eventually ask, "If you aren't vegetarian, why are you eating a vegetarian dish?" Rephrase what you would say instead of telling them, "Because I'm a vegan," and spiral into that social stigma conversation. Instead, tell them because you thought the dish would taste good or because you enjoy the taste of fried tofu versus the fried chicken they were offering. No one can argue with you if it is simply a matter of what your taste buds and stomach prefer at the moment, but someone will always argue with you over ideologies.

However, education on diet and lifestyle will be necessary at some point in time, especially if you ever want to talk about your eating habits with someone. Luckily, we have many popular myths in the next chapter that is easily and scientifically debunked to help begin your mental journey toward preparing for all aspects of your lifestyle, including the diet.

No one can argue with you if it is simply a matter of what your taste buds and stomach prefer at the moment, but someone will always argue with you over ideologies. However, education on diet and lifestyle will be necessary at some point in time, especially if you ever want to talk about your eating habits with someone. Luckily, we have many popular myths in the next chapter that is easily and scientifically debunked to help begin your mental journey toward preparing for all aspects of your lifestyle, including the diet.

Adopting a vegan lifestyle can help that statistic.

Chapter 2

Exposing The Myths

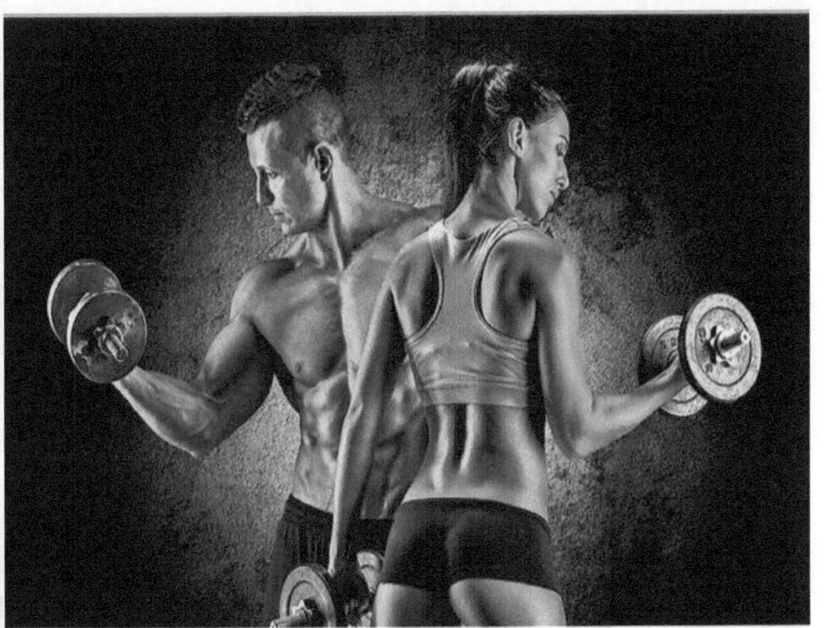

There are many different myths about the vegan community that perpetuate society. Some of them are large myths that have spread to the far corners of the world, and some of them are lesser-known myths that could wreak havoc on the community if the general public believes. We are here to introduce you to these myths before we completely debunk them.

Myth #1: Vegans don't get enough protein in their diets.

This is simply false. While meat, eggs, and milk are major protein sources, they are not the only ones. Many of our beloved vegetables have protein, like spinach. One cup of uncooked spinach has around 7 grams of protein. Nut butter has 8 grams of protein per two tablespoons, quinoa has around 9 grams per cup cooked, and one cup of cooked lentils packs a whopping 18 grams of protein! Many research studies have shown that vegans and traditional eaters usually get *too* much protein.

Myth #2: If you can't eat meat, then you can't build muscle to become strong.

There is so much false in this statement; it's unbelievable. Things like hemp powder and dairy-deprived whey protein sources pack incredible volumes of protein (just like those traditional protein shakes that bodybuilders belove), and the foods listed above are perfect meat protein "replacements" when it comes to taking in the required amount of protein to build and keep muscles strong. However, another myth also flows into this point as well: it is possible to get the recommended amount of calcium in a vegan diet without drinking, and eating dairy products will enable someone to keep muscles and bones healthy for the long term.

Raw nuts, calcium-fortified hemp milk, and cooked greens like broccoli and kale have great amounts of calcium per serving.

Myth #3: Vegans are weak.

First off, what? Secondly, no. NFL defensive lineman David Carter, 6-time Ironman champion John Joseph, and the tennis sisters Venus and Serena Williams are all vegans.

Need I say more?

Myth #4: Vegan diets are not healthy.

Suppose you've got me here if fruits, vegetables, non-GMO products, no MSG, and a lack of meat and dairy are unhealthy. However, I highly doubt that a diet oncologists recommend for certain cancer patients is unhealthy.

Not only does a vegan lifestyle afford the body more opportunities to acquire micro-and-macronutrients the body needs to operate and survive, but it also helps to flush out the toxins and free radicals that have built up within the body that have been deposited by over-processed foods, grain-fed animal meats, and even over-pasteurized dairy products.

Myth #5: You must supplement holes in your diet with vitamins if you go vegan, which will cost you more money.

Let's break down this one: supplements for holes in the diet. A vegan diet has been scientifically researched and measured against dozens of other diets, and it has come out on top time and time again as the most nutrient-dense diet on the planet. People who attempt a vegan lifestyle must supplement with vitamins because they cut out animal products and dairy. That is only half the battle. The other part is replacing those you have removed with things you can ingest.
This idea of supplements costing you money, which makes a vegan diet somehow unattainable because of the hit your pocketbook takes, is simply absurd. A basic multivitamin that houses between 30 and 60 once-a-day pills is between $12 and $15 U.S. dollars on the market. Would you like to tally how much you spend on takeout or fast food?

If you adopt a vegan lifestyle and remove animal products and dairy, you must ensure you replace those foods. Try other fruits and experiment with other vegetables! Try to broaden your taste buds, and as you do this, you will find other sources of vital nutrients and vitamins that were otherwise absent from your diet.

Myth #6: Veganism is an eating disorder.

No, no, no, no, and no. First, "veganism" is a lifestyle, while "vegan" is a way of eating. "Veganism" is a lifestyle that seeks to exclude all forms of animal cruelty and exploitation. This includes not eating animal products and byproducts, not purchasing clothing made from animal skins, and boycotting news and media outlets that either support or take no stance against animal cruelty.

"Vegan" is the eating lifestyle whereby animal products, byproducts, and dairy are removed from the diet and replaced with suitable fruits, vegetables, and fortified non-dairy products to maintain bodily health and promote a healthy lifestyle. An "eating disorder" is a mentally-based condition that surfaces in physical manifestations of control, resulting in an incredibly unhealthy treatment of the body.

Myth #7: Veganism is "white."

Some people believe that a vegan eating lifestyle and "veganism" in general is something that is only perpetrated and truly adopted in white upper-middle-class communities. Because of this, many people believe that vegans are somehow racist in nature, which is absolute and utter nonsense.

How do I know this? Well, refer back to myth #3. If you are unfamiliar with who any of those athletes are, we will sit back and wait for you to look them up quickly.

Myth #8: Vegans only eat vegetables, which taste horrendous.

Well, that's just insulting. Vegans eat all sorts of things, including vegetables. Raw nuts, all sorts of fruits, non-dairy fortified kinds of milk and drinks, freshly-squeezed juices, and hemp powder proteins are just a few foods vegans take in regularly. A "plant-based" diet is not a diet of salads; it is a diet of anything grown in plant form. This means potatoes, fresh herbs and spices, bananas, grapes, and virtually anything else that grows on a plant is consumable on this diet. These ingredients can make spicy bean chilies, hearty stews, sweet potato lasagnas, and even pizza!

Sounds pretty yummy to me.

The myths perpetrated in the public sector are usually myths concocted by the media. They swing stories for their benefit to garner ratings and attention without giving any thought to the detriment they are doing to society as a whole. Many people have been led away from adopting a vegan eating lifestyle because of things they have seen on the news that are not true. The myths above are just a handful perpetrated over the decades since plant-based diets have surged into the public eye, and it is important to understand that. However, if debunking these myths still have you wondering if you can stay physically fit in this eating lifestyle, then the next chapter is for you.

In the following chapter, we will outline many major athletes who have fully adopted a vegan eating lifestyle.

these myths are false and preposterous.

Chapter 3

Vegan Competitors with Strength

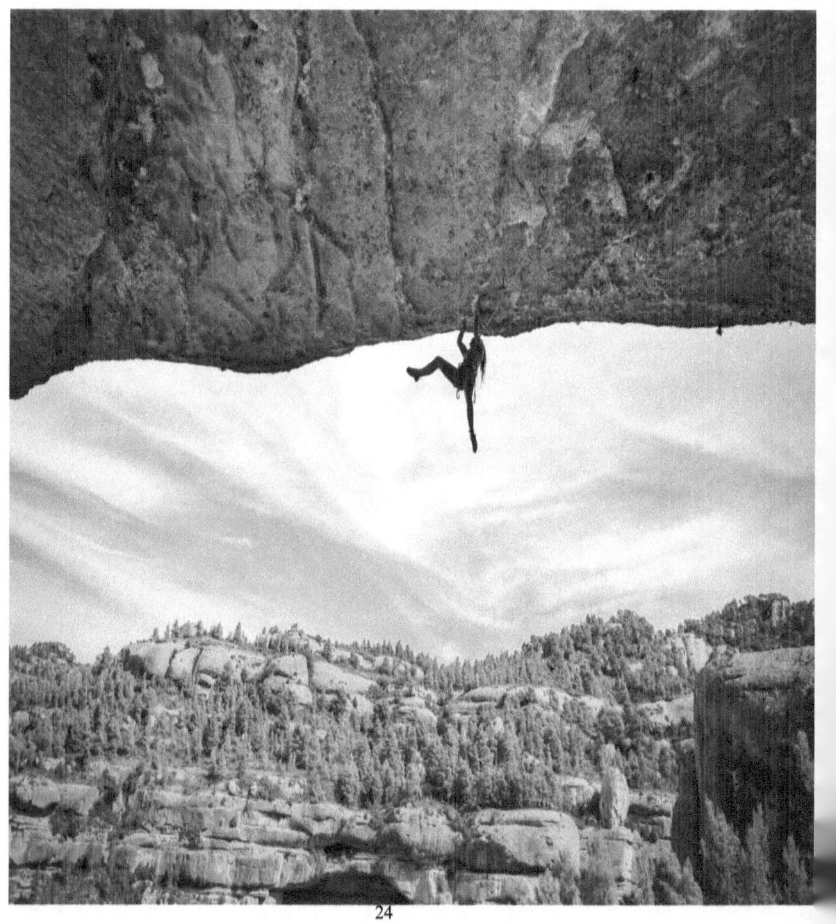

Many prominent athletes have adopted vegan diets and lifestyles. They have maintained their strength and promoted their inward health past a point they felt possible as a traditional eater.

Venus Williams

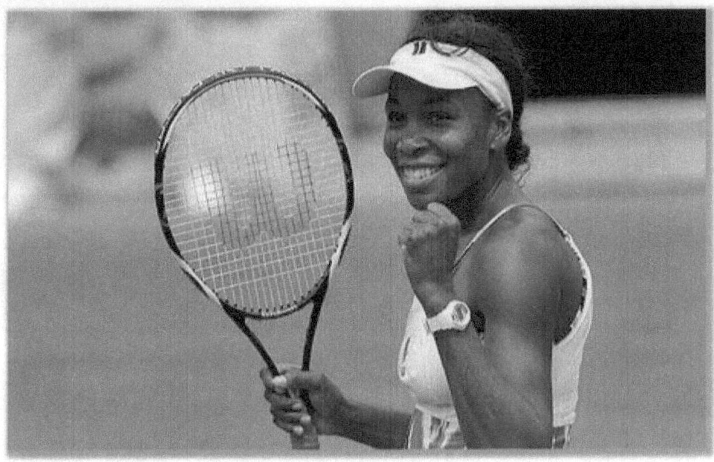

One of the most infamous stories is, of course, Venus Williams. In 2011, Venus was diagnosed with Sjogren's syndrome, which is an autoimmune disease, and this is what prompted her to adopt a raw vegan lifestyle. When her diagnosis took her out of the world of tennis, adopting this eating lifestyle brought her back to the court despite her autoimmune condition. Ever since, she has trained harder, become more efficient, and has stood alongside her sister (who also adopted the vegan lifestyle to support her sister through this uncertain road) and has since stood toe-to-toe with her on the court.

Mike Tyson

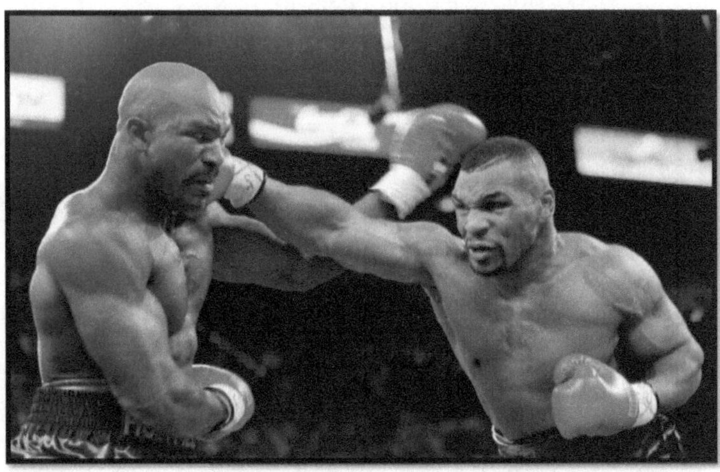

Mike Tyson is another athlete who has stayed strong and kept his muscle mass even after switching to a plant-based diet. When Tyson made the switch to clean living, he became an outspoken proponent of the vegan lifestyle. He dropped over 100 pounds after cutting meat and animal byproducts from his diet, and he proclaims that it has helped him with various issues he began experiencing as he got older. He tells anyone who will listen that as his age starts to creep up; he felt his physical condition slipping.

He was experiencing arthritis, sharp joint pain, and tacking on weight at an enormous rate. Since switching to plant-based eating and an animal-free lifestyle, not only have those issues cleared up, but he has also gained the bulk of his energy back in the latter years of his life.

Mac Danzig

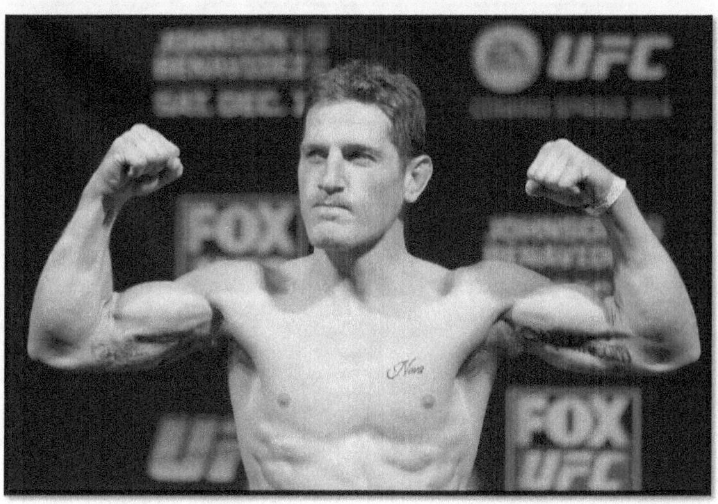

Mac Danzig is a prominent name in the world of MMA fighting, and he was criticized a great deal when he decided to adopt a plant-based diet. In the meat-eating world of MMA, he now stuck out like a sore thumb. While he cut dairy out quite sometime before the full move because of allergies, he states that he shifted to a full-on plant-based diet because he felt his body was not at the peak physical condition it could have been regarding his fighting.

A prominent MMA fighter adopted a plant-based eating regimen because he *wanted more from his body.*

Among the foods he eats regularly are black beans, lentils, and seeds.

Hank Aaron

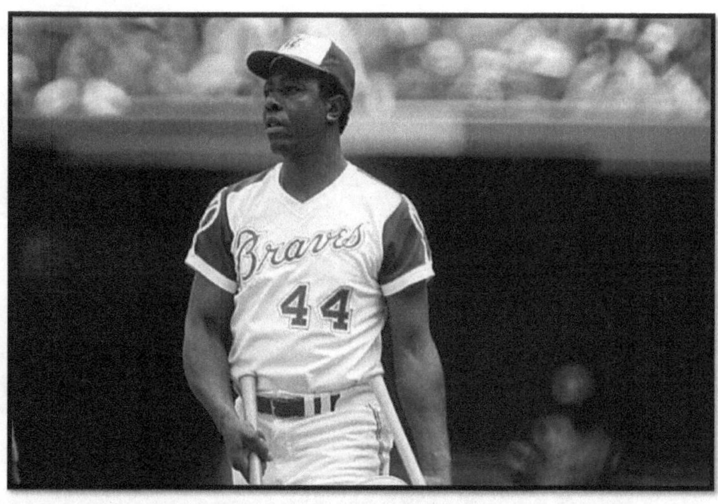

Baseball superstar Hank Aaron is just another prominent athlete in the world of athletes that adopted a plant-based lifestyle to further their strength, agility, and energy stores for their career. He is a 25-time All-Star in baseball and has never argued or disputed his diet with the press. Simply the length of his illustrious and historical career tells us that a plant-based lifestyle is good for the body and shows that it has no bearing on an individual's strength.

Tony Gonzalez

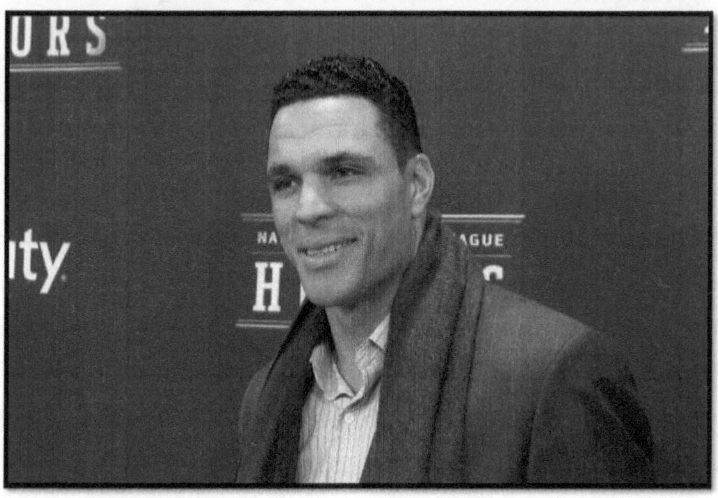

However, no list of vegan athletes is complete without the mention of Tony Gonzalez. An infamous tight end in the NFL, he has openly admitted that his dietary choices have caused many awkward eyebrows raises during his career. The catalyst for his decision was a meeting he had on an airplane with businessman David Pulaski.

What happened during that encounter? Well, Pulaski kept refusing standard meat-and-cheese dishes offered to first-class passengers on the plane they were both inhabiting, and Gonzalez got curious and asked why.

Pulaski introduced him to The China Study, an experiment where multiple scientists found that Chinese citizens who ate fewer animal products were less susceptible to many illnesses. Pulaski talked with him about the theories behind many illnesses that plague Americans regarding their diets, and the rest is history.

Gonzalez is the billboard example of a vegan diet's dangers and benefits. When he first began his diet, he dropped a substantial amount of weight because he was uninformed about the nutrition side of the eating lifestyle.

In essence? He cut out all animal products without replacing them with other protein, fruit, and vegetable sources.

Due to this weight loss, he lost his strength, so he began educating himself. He spoke with several doctors and specialists, read every material he could get his hands on, figured out where he had gone wrong, and made every effort to change it. He quickly began incorporating more plant protein sources he didn't know existed, putting him back in fighting shape within a few short months.

So, what has this plant-based diet done for his career? Well, since adopting the diet, he has not only become incredibly outspoken about his decisions because of the criticism many in the NFL gave him (which has led many individuals to adopt vegan eating habits of their own), but he has also set several athletic records within his career, including a career reception record for his position in football.

The truth is that adopting a plant-based lifestyle if done right and with the right amount of knowledge, can help your body heal. Not only that, but it can also help to strengthen your body in ways a traditional eating lifestyle cannot because the variety of foods you have to adopt will also come jampacked with macro-and-micronutrients your body is not getting otherwise.

So, with all of this in mind, what does a vegan eat? Do they take supplements anyway? What foods have those sources of protein and calcium that are vital to bone and muscle health?

Trust me; there is more variety than you realize.

CHAPTER 4
HOW DO YOU FUEL THE VEGAN ATHLETE?

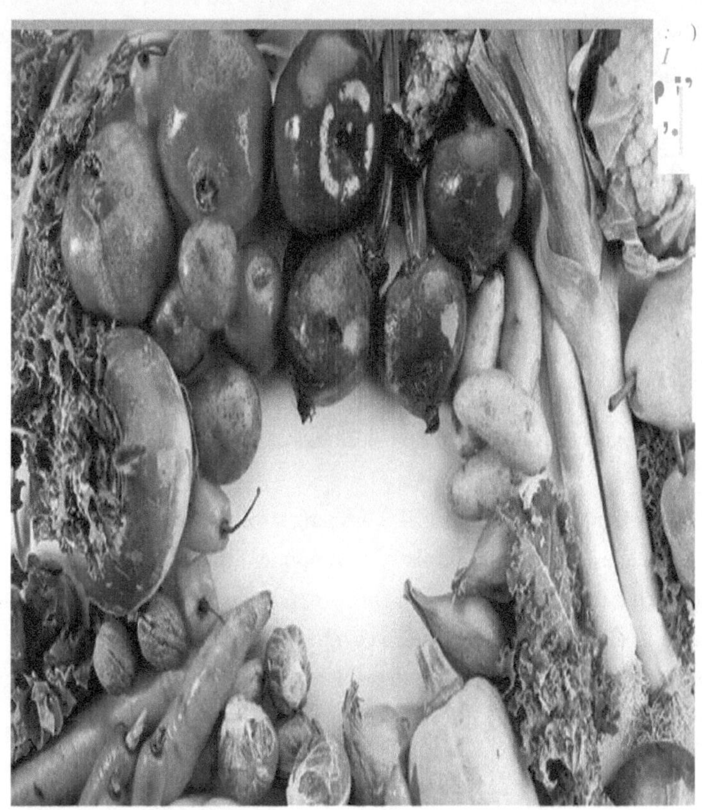

A vegan lifestyle includes ingesting fruits, vegetables, grains, dried beans, peas, lentils, seeds, and nuts. Vegans do not consume dairy, eggs, meat, poultry, fish, or any products containing these foods. Many people struggle with adopting a vegan lifestyle because they believe deficiencies in calcium, iron, zinc, and other vital vitamins and nutrients will occur. And, in part, they are right... if they do not replace what they have removed with other sources of these vitamins and minerals.

Suppose a traditional eater removes all dairy and animal products from their diet and regularly eats despite that removal. In that case, they will be deficient in vitamins, minerals, protein, and caloric intake.

Vegan Sources of Macro-and-Micro-Nutrients

There are plenty of vegan sources of these very important macro- and-micro-nutrients you can place into your diet once removing dairy and animal byproducts to "plug the holes" those food items will cause.

Protein is vital to building muscle, keeping strong, and ensuring red blood cells are healthy. It is also the component that supports growth throughout a species' life cycle. Sources of protein for vegans include soy and soy-based products (such as tempeh, fortified soy beverages, and tofu), veggie burgers, legumes (black beans, kidney beans, black-eyed peas, and lentils), grains (quinoa, oatmeal, and brown rice), seeds (sunflower and sesame) and nut butter.

Iron is another vital component of a healthy diet because it helps carry oxygen to different parts of the body. It is said that vegans usually need twice the amount of iron in their diet as traditional eaters because these iron sources from plants are not as well-absorbed as the iron from animal foods, but that does not mean a vegan eating lifestyle is bad. The foods that contain iron also contain high amounts of micronutrients that most all other people are consistently deficient in.

Sources for iron include soy and soy-based products, veggie burgers, prune juice, dried apricots, cooked spinach, cooked kale, potatoes with the skin on, pinto beans, adzuki beans, lentils, fortified grain products, cashews, almonds, blackstrap molasses.

One thing to remember about absorbing iron while eating vegan is that it absorbs better when ingested with foods rich in vitamin C. These foods include grapefruits, oranges, kiwis, lemons, limes, potatoes, sweet peppers, broccoli, and cantaloupe. And yes, their juices also count if you are a juicer.

Vitamin B12 is yet another vitamin that many would be deficient in if they did not replace those foods removed from their diet. This vitamin helps the body utilize stored fats and create red blood cells.

Good sources of vitamin B12 for a vegan include Red Star nutritional yeast, fortified soy beverages, and fortified meat alternatives like meatless chicken and veggie burgers.

Vitamin D is necessary for the body because it not only helps to stave off seasonal depression and help regulate the brain's chemistry, but it also aids in the absorption and converts phosphorus and calcium into usable components that aid in strong teeth and bones. Vegan sources of vitamin D include non-hydrogenated kinds of margarine and fortified, vegan-friendly products.

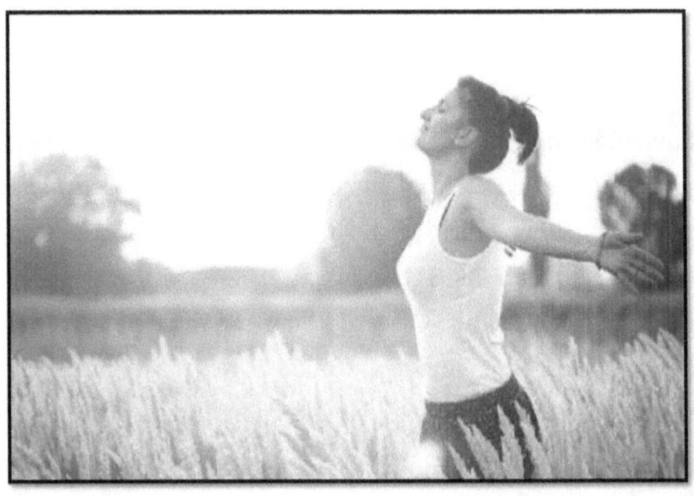

Also, the sun. Get outside and get yourself some sun.

Speaking of calcium, that is another one of the controversial nutrients that vegans supposedly do not get enough of. Calcium is necessary for bone and muscle health and helps with muscular contractions as your heart beats. There are numerous calcium sources for vegans: soy yogurt, fortified non-dairy beverages, navy beans, sesame butter (also called "tahini"), blackstrap molasses, bok choy, okra, figs, and fortified orange juice.

Zinc is another mineral many people are deficient in, and there are many sources of it for those who choose a vegan eating lifestyle. Zinc is necessary for basic development and growth, and it also aids in strengthening the immune system and healing wounds inflicted upon the body.

Good sources of zinc for vegans include peas, lentils, dried beans, pecans, cashew butter, peanut butter, pumpkin seeds, and fortified whole grains.

The last nutrient many people lack that can be provided for on a vegan diet is linolenic acid. If you do not recognize that name, you will probably recognize it by its other name, omega-3 fatty acid. Omega-3s are important for nerve, eye, and brain development but are also helpful in preventing heart disease and cardiac events. Some wonderful vegan-friendly sources include flaxseed, soybean, canola, ground flaxseed, tofu, and walnuts.

When To Take Supplement?

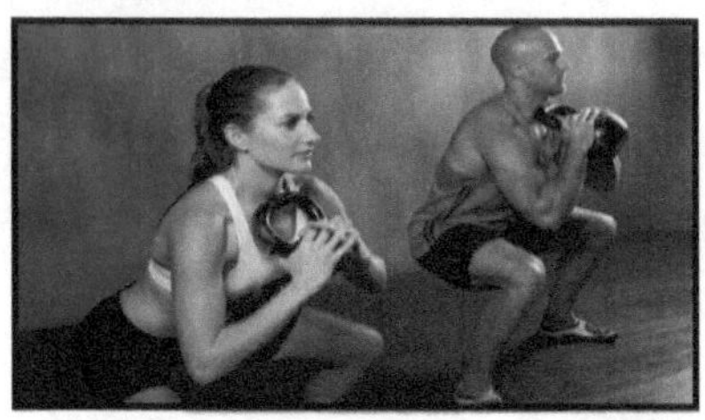

But supplements are usually something if you are an athlete or work out intensively while adopting a vegan lifestyle.

Worked into the health regimen, no matter what. Vegans, however, must be very careful with the types of supplements they take. Many supplements on the market have animal byproduct additives to aid their preservation and shelf-life. It can wreak havoc on a vegan's body if they have gone without consuming animal products or byproducts for an extended period.

If you find yourself a picky eater, then all of the nutrients and vitamins listed above would be wonderful to work into your morning or evening routine. Just make sure you find a vegan-friendly distributor of these vitamins to stay within the boundaries of your diet.

A basic vegan-certified multivitamin that includes B12 will be enough for most vegans. Those multivitamins house zinc, iodine, vitamin C, omega-3 fatty acids, and a slew of micronutrients your body can benefit from. However, suppose you are eating a vegan lifestyle and training or working out regularly. In that case, it is recommended that you find a vegan-friendly branched-chain amino acid to help your body recuperate from the beating your muscles are taking in your workout sessions. These BCAA's will help your body maintain the muscles it breaks down and strengthens instead of losing your strength. It will also aid in keeping your bones strong during training, as well.

The truth is that dropping entire food groups from your body, while healthier, will inevitably create holes in the nutrients you receive. Our stereotypical dietary pyramid that kids are taught in school is not focused on keeping their body inwardly healthy for the long run but is there to ensure they get the right amount of vitamins and minerals daily.

In other words, our dietary pyramid is not constructed with bodily health but with nutrient health in mind.

And yes, there is a difference. This means that supplements will be necessary. How will you know if you need supplements? Start by finding a basic vegan-friendly multivitamin you can take daily (and a vegan-friendly BCAA if you are working out and training regularly), and see how your body feels from there.

If there is a list outlined above whose foods you cannot stomach, then that is an individual nutrient and/or vitamin that will probably require its bulk daily supplement. But now that you have all of this information, it is time to tackle the last informational part of this book before we talk about "going vegan" and what it entails. This last part addresses the intimidating work of exercise and what it means and looks like to someone who eats a vegan diet.

CHAPTER 5

IS THERE A VEGAN WORKOUT PLAN?

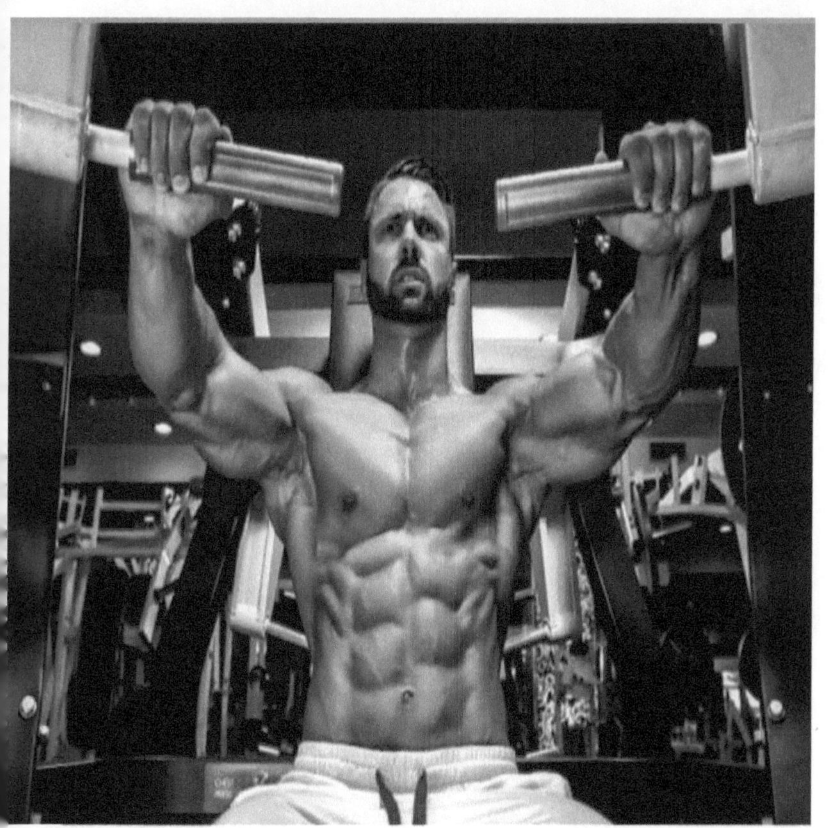

Getting and becoming active can be difficult for many people regardless of diet. A lack of motivation, morbid obesity, time restraints, and other issues make it very easy for people to either not have the time or not find the energy to become motivated to move. Each person has a unique case, and no single solution fits everyone. However, if you have chosen to adopt a vegan diet, then you have already taken one step in the right direction for the health of your body for the long term.

This means the next major step will be figuring out what workout plan you want to utilize.

Beginning the plan

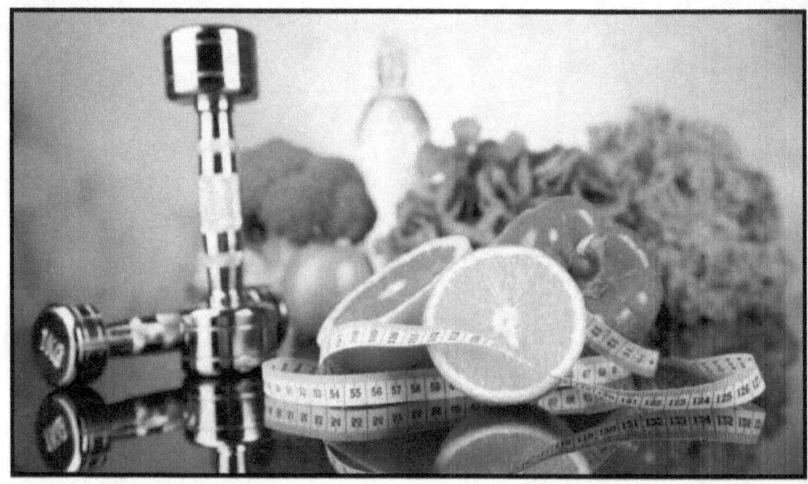

A common way for beginners to exercise is to take an easy start. This usually means going outside and walking short 10-minute bursts or taking the plunge to get that gym membership and going and walking on a treadmill for 15 minutes. You can do particular exercises in your home for people who want to do some muscle training.

Another important facet is keeping motivated during your exercise. The most popular way people keep motivated is via music, but you can also utilize television to help you develop the habit of regular exercise. The whole point of beginning an exercise journey on a vegan diet is to make sure to ingrain the habit.

To complete your path in your journey towards better health, you have to choose a workout plan. This will be a plan you follow week-by-week that can be easily tailored upwards as your body becomes more efficient in utilizing its energy and becomes generally stronger. Even though you are eating a vegan lifestyle, all of your muscle groups in some way need to be exercised. This includes your abdomen, thighs, and back and arms muscles. Simply doing nothing but cardio will not make you stronger, and it is not an efficient use of the calories you give your body.

Tips For Vegans

People have to keep in mind when exercising on a vegan diet that you will have to feed your body more to keep up your energy. Traditional eaters consume massive amounts of protein, indicative of the size of their workout program because protein from animal sources stays in the body longer, an individual who eats meat and animal byproducts could go to a restaurant and have a nice meal, then still have that fuel two hours later when they decide to go to the gym.

Vegans do not have that kind of convenience.

Because plant-based protein sources are not as easily absorbed into the body, nor are they held onto for as long as meat-based protein sources, some energy must be given to the body within 30 minutes of the exercise you choose to do.

Not only that, but you usually have to replenish that store of energy after your workout. This does not mean you must eat an entire meal before and after your workout. This means that a snack, a juice, or a shake should be ingested 30 minutes before and no later than 30 minutes after your workout.

The Cardio Guidelines

Cardio is an imperative part of a workout regimen for a vegan because it will help keep your blood sugars at bay with the number of carbohydrates you will take in on this diet. The thing about a vegan diet is that even though it eliminates food groups, it does not designate a specific amount of caloric or carbohydrate intake that has to be eaten throughout the day. So, cardio and all of its offshoots will help individuals regulate their blood sugars when figuring out the appropriate caloric intake for their body.

Things like 15-minute walks outside, 15-minute walks on the treadmill, 30 minutes of swimming, cycling classes, and even
yoga videos you can do in the comfort of your own home all count as legitimate sources of cardio you should implement at least three times a week.

Strength Training

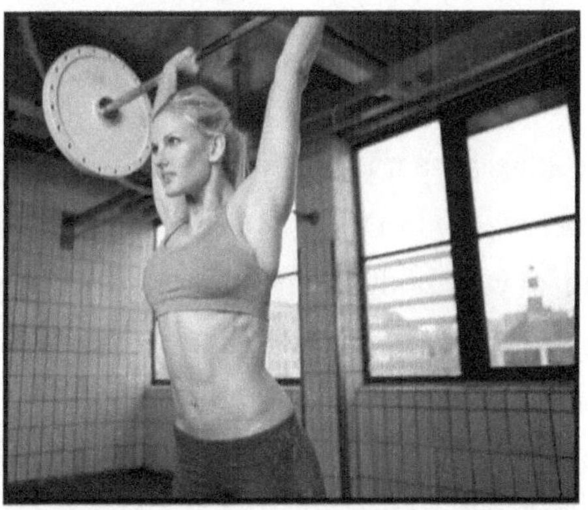

Strength training for your muscles and your bones also needs to be incorporated into your workout, and it should be between 30 and 45 minutes each time you go to do it. The reason why you do not
want to go over 45 minutes because it can be over-exhausting to the muscle groups you are working with and can cause damage that will

keep you from exercising. You do not want to hit all of the muscle groups more than twice a week because this will also ensure that you keep an even muscle development over all of the muscles of your body without overworking and hurting yourself.

For those just beginning their strength training, you can do simple weightlifting in the comfort of your own home. You can also do bodyweight squats and calf raises to work the lower half of your body. Push-ups and sit-ups will work your arms, upper back, and abdomen; planks are a great way to engage all of the body's muscles.

And they can *all* be done in the comfort of your own home.

Strength training is a little more fluid in how often to implement it throughout the week because it is less tailored to the number of times you "do it" and more tailored to the number of times you have worked out a specific group of your body. Remember: during the week for strength training, you have to work every muscle of your body *twice*. Whether you situate it so you are strength training every day, or whether you situate it so you are strength training three times a week, it does not matter. What matters is the length of time you train strength and the duration you touch on those major muscle groups weekly.

Alternative Workout Plans

There are other ways to incorporate working out into your lifestyle that is less traditional and more convenient for familial lifestyles. Sports, climbing a tree with your kids or
your family, gymnastics, and resistance bands are wonderful ways to enhance your workout plan without stepping into a gym. There are also certain classes you can take out in the community that has the potential to get you around many other like-minded individuals, such as martial arts and kickboxing. These avenues are great because they incorporate cardio and strength training and enhance your bones' strength.

Now, it is time for the most important chapter in this book. Up until this point, you have merely been fed information. You have been instructed on the guidelines that eating a vegan diet affords, you have been instructed on the types of exercising you can implement, and you have even seen us debunk multiple myths that come with the vegan diet that society has misinterpreted and perpetuated.
It is time to go over how to correctly and safely implement this change in your life so you have the greatest chance of succeeding.

CHAPTER 6

TIPS FOR STARTING YOUR VEGAN LIFESTYLE

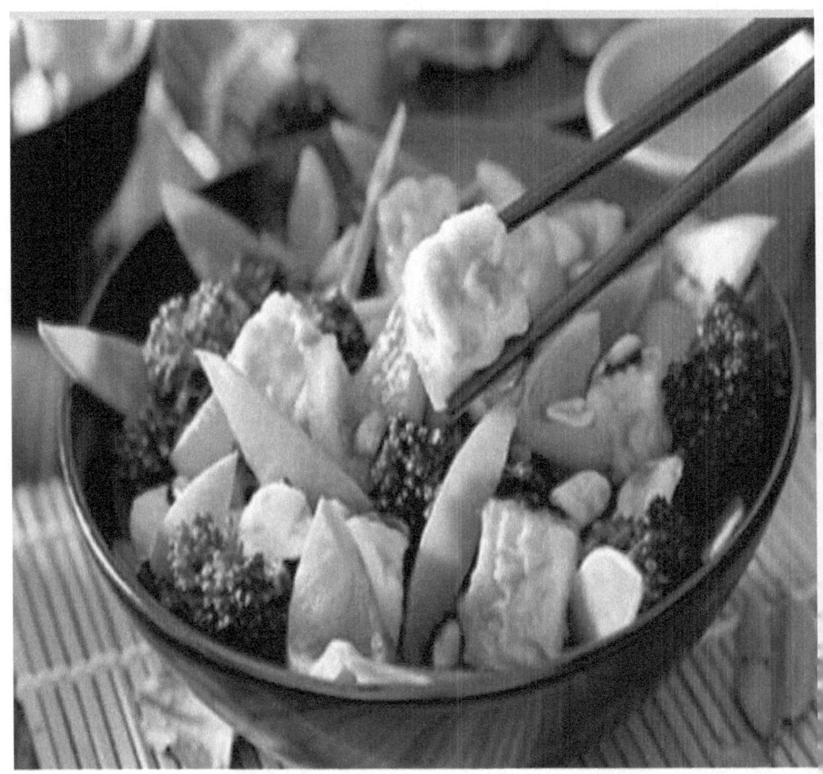

The first step for any new lifestyle change is to do your research. However, we have already done the heavy lifting for you. So! You have decided to take the plunge into a vegan way of eating. You have cleared out your home of all animal products and byproducts and filled your home with lots of things according to the food list outlined above.

Now what?

Go Vegan, Not Famishment!

Understand one thing: your body is not supposed to be hungry. Suppose you give your body ample amounts of healthy foods filled with nutrients. In that case, you will lose weight easily. 4,000 calories of fast food and 4,000 calories of fresh fruits, vegetables, and legumes are completely different. Your body will lose weight by instilling the latter rather than the former. Do not think that adopting a vegan diet to lose weight or help your long-term health means going hungry.

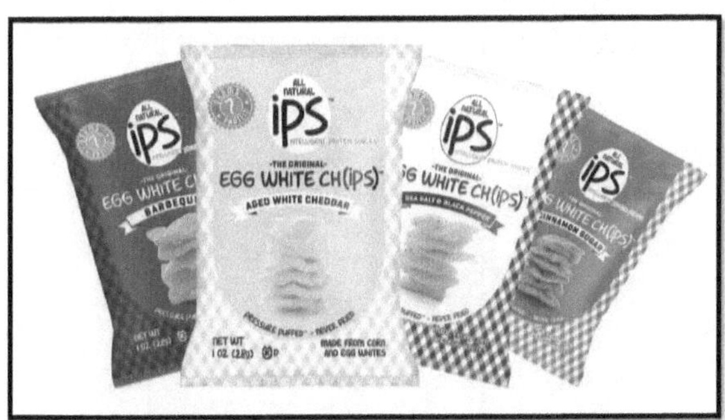

Grab a snack if you get hungry in between meals.

Listen To Your Body

Awareness is also a vital part of "going vegan." Listening to your body and interpreting what it wants is imperative to giving it the nutrients it longs for daily. For most people, it is easy to distinguish between when the body is thirsty and when it is hungry. However, for many of those "other people," it can be hard when the body becomes hungry but has no particular craving. Becoming in tune with your body and interpreting its needs via the brain signals being shot throughout your system is vital to becoming a vegan.

Not only that, it is vital to becoming a well-adjusted individual.

Tips For Long-Term Lifestyle Change

For many, implementing a lifestyle is not something you can "do." As in, jumping in feet first will always lead them down a path of failure. If you can throw out or donate all the food in your kitchen, refill it, and start your new eating lifestyle full-force tomorrow, you are more likely to succeed.

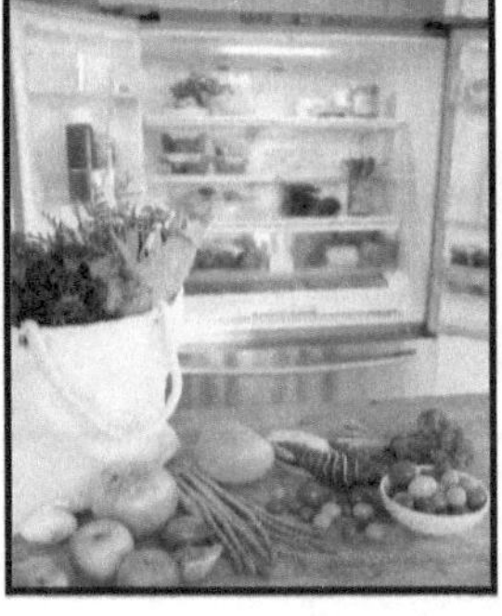

But not everyone is like that.

For those who are not like that, you can go through your kitchen and take stock of everything that will not be kosher for a vegan-eating lifestyle. All meats, refined sugars, snacks, and animal byproducts need to be written down on this list, and then you need to put this list somewhere where you will see it every day.

Every time you go grocery shopping, cross two items off that list that you will not purchase and refill your kitchen with and, instead, replace them with something for your new plant-based diet

that you will regularly incorporate into your kitchen. For example, if you are ditching the chips and salsa, opt for something crunchy, like carrots, and then purchase all the ingredients needed to make your salsa!

Another tip is to eat before you go shopping. If you go into a grocery store hungry, sticking with your vegan shopping list will be much harder if you constantly pass the junk food and candy aisles. It will also behoove you, at least for the first few trips, to write your grocery list and take it with you. Whether you jot it down on your phone or write it out physically on paper, having that accountability right in front of you will help you stay on track.

Making these small changes in your diet will help you instill the diet for the long haul, resulting in long-term health advances that will not only help you lose weight but will help advance the efficiency of your body and heal your organs and immune system. Adapting to a diet change like this takes time, so take it in stride. Understand that 70% of this process is mental, and overcoming those mental barriers will help you reach a point where a vegan lifestyle is not simply a "diet" but a new way of life.

Some daily habits you can begin implementing are making up snacks before wanting them, meal-planning your week,

designating one day a week to grocery shop, and always keep trying new foods and learning. Making your snacks before wanting them will help keep you from jeopardizing your new way of eating by grabbing something more convenient and meal-planning your week will help keep you from falling prey to the convenience of take-out.

Not only that but designating one day a week to grocery shop will help your wallet because you can use all the fresh products you purchased before it wilts and goes bad. A vegan diet is easier on your wallet if you can minimize food waste by shopping every week instead of every paycheck.

Feed Your Mind

But the most important thing is always to keep learning. Purchase a book on the vegan diet every so often and read through it to see if there is any new information. Research exotic fruits and vegetables you can try at that new restaurant that has opened up downtown. Research and listen to other athletes and prominent vegan individuals to see what works for them.

Like any other way of eating, veganism and the vegan diet are not static entities. Eating the same things day in and day out without ever trying new things or implementing new tactics is going to get boring.

Not only that, it can create massive nutritional holes in your diet.

Stick to these steps and habits necessary for implementing a vegan diet. You are well on your way to improving your long-term health, losing weight, aiding the environment, and even tapping into a store of strength and energy you did not realize you could have.

Becoming a vegan is about strength, mental acuity, and determination. It takes dedication and knowledge to properly and healthfully enact a vegan lifestyle, so make sure you never stop learning about the diet and all it entails.

There are many myths floating around out there that misappropriate and perpetuate false information when it comes to a vegan lifestyle. If you are nervous about taking supplements, then understand this: traditional eaters are the biggest consumers of supplements on the market.

Why?

Because despite them eating animal products and byproducts, they are still deficient in their intake of vitamins and minerals because of a massive reduction in fruits and vegetables. Many traditional eaters are under the assumption that animal products and byproducts will give them everything they need is not true. Traditional eaters usually consume too much protein and drain their energy stores because of a lack of proper nutrition.

Yes, becoming a vegan in terms of diet and lifestyle helps the environment, but that is not the only reason to adopt this diet. Several research studies that have been conducted have paired a vegan diet against many other diets, such as vegetarian, traditional diet, a low-carbohydrate diet, high-fat diet, and even high-protein diets.
Not only did participants in a vegan diet lose 9.3 more pounds on average than any other person on any other diet tested, but they also saw a drastic balancing of their blood sugar levels, heart rate, and blood pressure.
Do not allow anyone to convince you that "going vegan" will somehow ruin your strength. The Williams sisters, professional NFL football players, boxers, and even MMA athletes are just a few among the thousands of athletes who eat a plant-based diet. Many of those athletes have discovered strength they did not know they had and have told people time and time again that they would never have unlocked that strength and fortitude if they had not adopted a plant-based eating lifestyle.

Protein is not the end-all-be-all of strength. It takes massive amounts of micro- and-macronutrients to upkeep your muscles and bones at a cellular level. A diverse vegan diet gives you plenty of those to stay healthy in the gym. All those micro-and-macronutrients also afford you more energy, so recuperation from the gym and any other workout regimen will be quicker.

Exercise is something you need to implement on a vegan diet. Whether you take a walk for 15 minutes every day or you begin your journey down a 2-hour workout regimen to build and tone muscle, you need to make sure two things occur: you need to make sure it is a steady plan you can handle, and you need to make sure all of the facets of your health are being exercised. What this means is that just cardio or just weight-lifting is not going to work. There has to be a healthy combination of both to succeed at exercising while adopting a vegan eating lifestyle.

Bonus Section

The most popular way to adopt this is to work out six times a week, with three days being cardio-based and three days being muscle-based. That cardio can range anywhere from a walk around your block to swimming for an hour, and that strength training can range anywhere from doing sit-ups and pushups in your own home to going to the gym and utilizing their weight machines.

Whatever you choose to do, and whatever you find works for you, stick to it.

I hope this book educated you and helped you to feel more comfortable with the idea of eating vegan.

The next step is to implement! Whether you take it one step at a time or you start full-throttle tomorrow, the next step is physical implementation. And I promise you, you can do this. You are stronger than you realize

Veganism is a concept that deals with abstaining from the consumption of animal-based products such as milk, eggs, and meat. Vegans follow a strict vegetarian diet minus dairy products. Vegans can only consume vegetables, fruits, grains, legumes, nuts, and seeds.

This does not sound like an ideal diet for athletes, as most rely on animal protein, like meats and eggs, to develop a strong body. However, the world of veganism can offer several superfoods that are great for developing a strong body and can increase an athlete's vitality.

If you are a vegan athlete, you have come to the right place, as we will look at seven superfoods that can be incorporated into your daily diet.

Let's begin!

7 SUPERFOODS FOR VEGAN ATHLETES

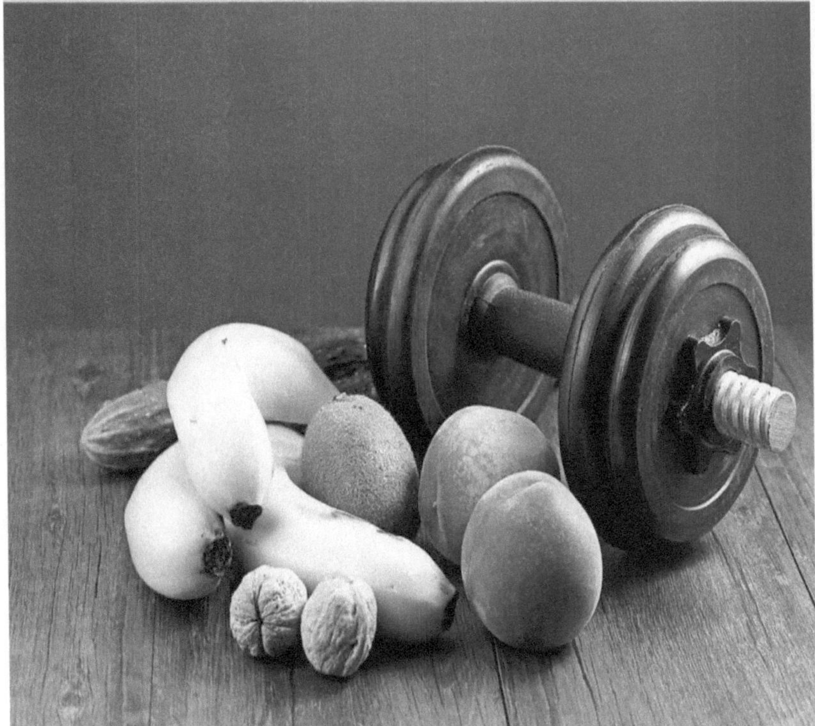

Berries

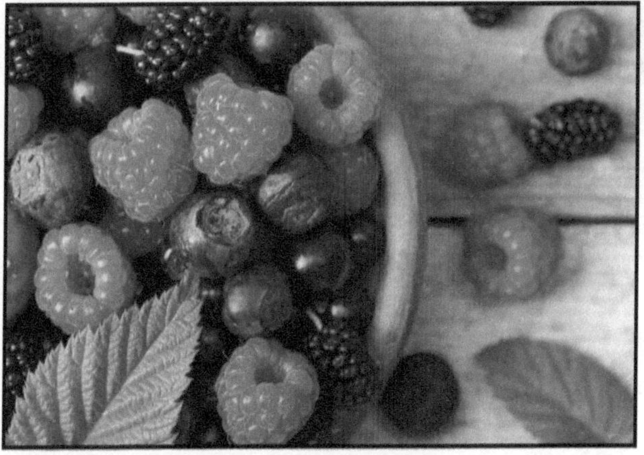

Kick-starting the list of vegan superfoods are berries! Berries are one of the most recommended foods for athletes and for a good reason. Berries can offer the body several benefits that are highlighted as shown below:

Muscle recovery

Berries are credited for increasing muscle recovery. They help reduce your body's recovery from muscle tears and soreness. According to an experiment conducted on athletes, where they were given blueberry smoothies
before their workout, they recovered better from muscle soreness 60 hours after their session.

Oxidative stress

The same experiment also found that berries greatly reduced oxidative stress as blood samples drawn 60 hours post-workout showed less cell damage. An athlete releases more free radicals into the body after a workout session. Being rich in antioxidants, Berries have the power to reverse oxidative damage to a large extent. This is quite important when it comes to maintaining not just muscle health but overall wellness.

Fat cell development

Berries help in inhibiting fat cell development. Fat cells must be controlled to prevent fat deposits from accumulating in the body. As per studies conducted on mice, those chewed on polyphenols- a nutrient in berries- saw a 73% decrease in lipids. This shows that berries can help cur curb fat deposits in the body.

Metabolic syndrome

Berries are said to help in the fight against metabolic syndrome. This syndrome can induce reduced metabolism, inflammation, glucose intolerance, insulin resistance, etc. Those who cannot exercise long hours will see a marked improvement in their stamina after consuming berries.

Here are some berries to add to your daily diet:

Acai berry

Being rich in antioxidant properties, Acai berries are great for athletes. Most athletes suffer from immense pain after a workout due to lactic acid buildup. Berries help in cutting down on this acid, thereby reducing the pain.

Blueberries

Blueberries are the king of berries and are a must for all athletes to include in their diet. Blueberries have extreme anti-oxidant content and a chemical known as Lactate dehydrogenase that helps reduce oxidative damage. This, in turn, helps enhance muscle health and helps athletes recover faster from muscle tears and soreness.

Goji berries

Goji berries help in increasing cellular respiration. This means your cells will have more oxygen before and after a workout, enabling better performance. These berries also contain Lactate dehydrogenase, making them a must-have in your diet.

As you can see, nibbling on a few berries before and after your workout can help in increasing your athletic performance to a large extent.

Oatmeal

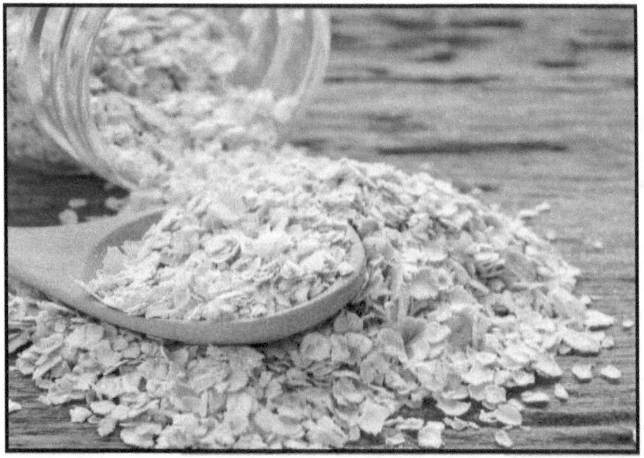

It is no secret that oatmeal is considered to be a favorite breakfast all over the world. It keeps you full and provides your body with lots of fiber. However, these are just minor benefits compared to the ones they can provide athletes.

Oatmeal is quite a popular ingredient in a bodybuilder's diet and is an important component of daily meals. It need not always be consumed for breakfast and can be eaten as a pre/post-workout snack. Here are some of the reasons that make oatmeal ideal for athletes.

B vitamins

One important vitamin that is essential for the upkeep of muscle health and metabolism is B vitamin. B vitamins include vitamins B6, B7, B3, and B5, all required to improve muscle function. A cup of oats can give your body the requisite B vitamins and increase muscle recovery. You will also feel energetic for several hours without having to snack.

Magnesium

An important component of an athlete's diet is magnesium. Magnesium is required to relieve sore muscles, enhance cell repair and cut down on the stress hormone known as cortisol. Magnesium also helps in maintaining a healthy nervous system. A single cup of cooked oats can leave you with 275 milligrams of magnesium, much more than several vegan foods combined can offer.

Proteins

It's a no-brainer that athletes require proteins to build stronger muscles. Proteins help build leaner muscles that are not easily burned away during the performance. People might wonder how vegans can meet this protein requirement without the addition of meats and eggs to their diet. The answer lies in oatmeal, as they can easily replace these ingredients and increase body proteins by a large margin. Just ½ a cup of cooked oats can contain 7 to 9 grams of proteins, which is ideal for athletes. Dry oats are often added to pre-post-workout shakes to capitalize on their protein content.

Iron

An athlete's body requires a good dose of iron, as it binds with oxygen and circulates throughout the body. A cup of cooked oats can provide 18% of the minimum requirement, making it a must-have in the mornings.

Beta-glucans

No athlete's diet will be complete without the addition of foods that are rich in beta-glucans. These help drain cholesterol from the bloodstream and provide the body with ample soluble fibers. You will have the chance to develop a leaner waistline through the consumption of oatmeal regularly.

You can prepare oats using water or substitute milk with almond or soymilk as a vegan.

Leafy greens (Kale and spinach)

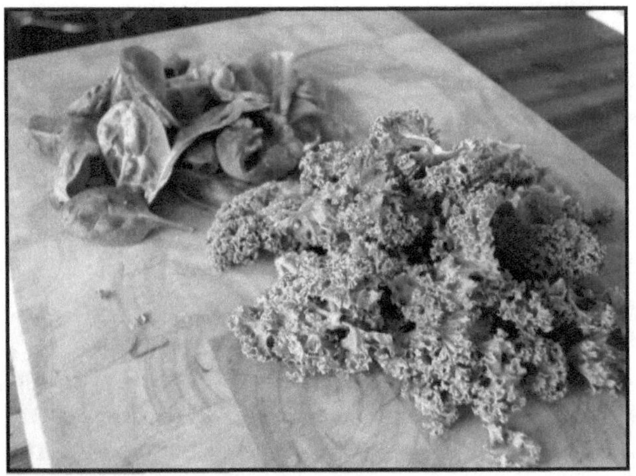

Leafy green vegetables are loaded with multiple vitamins required to maintain a healthy body. One can choose from several leafy green vegetables, but kale and spinach take top billing for their amazing health benefits. Some of these benefits are as follows.

* Kale

Nutrients

Kale is rich in many essential nutrients, including iron, Vitamins A, C, and K. These help increase your body's capacity to recover from muscle soreness. It also contains the highest amount of lutein, which is a potent antioxidant. Kale assists in enhancing cell repair and ensures that your body has the chance to recover after each session fully.

Cholesterol

No athlete can resist digging into some of their favorite snacks. This includes potato chips and wafers that athletes tend to eat, feeling guilty. However, one great substitute for this can be baked kale chips. They taste great and ensure you do not consume unnecessary calories and cholesterol. Kale is known to reduce cholesterol levels in your bloodstream, making it the best snacking option for vegan athletes.

- Spinach

Calories

Spinach is low in calorie content. Spinach can be quite filling without the addition of unwanted calories. Just a quick blitz in the blender, and you are left with a healthy juice sure to increase your nutrition through several folds.

Energy

Spinach is said to contain nitrates that contribute toward increasing cellular efficiency. You will feel energetic before and after a workout and have enough energy to carry on without feeling too tired.

Bones

It is crucial for athletes, especially women athletes, to pay keen attention to their bone health. Excessive pressure on bones during workouts and performance can weaken them and lead to bone deficiencies. One good way of dealing with this is through the incorporation of spinach into your day-to-day diet. Spinach contains abundant vitamin K, which is required to maintain strong bones. It also contains calcium that can further improve bone health.

Fiber

Fiber is required to digest food and maintain a clean stomach. Spinach can provide you with a good dose of fiber. Just a cup of spinach juice will leave you with 3 to 4 grams of fiber.

Apart from kale and spinach, you can also consume arugula, chard, collard greens, curly endive, and tatsoi.

Nuts (Walnuts and Almonds)

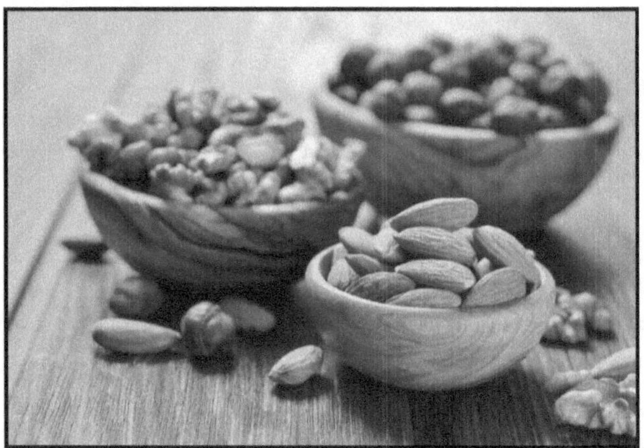

Walnuts are nutritional powerhouses designed to keep your body strong and healthy. A handful of walnuts increase your overall health and make you a better athlete.

- Walnuts

Here are why walnuts make for an athlete's best friend.

Amino acid

Amino acids are required for the upkeep of cells and muscles. It forms a large part of our body's cell structure. Walnuts contain an amino acid known as L-arginine, which is required to maintain muscle health. This amino acid converts to nitric oxide, a compound that causes blood vessels to dilate. This improves blood flow to the various muscles and reduces the risk of tearing.

Omega 3 fatty acids

Walnuts consist of omega-3 fatty acids that are required to maintain heart health. It reduces inflammation and helps with the conversion of fat to energy. Walnuts are regarded as the number 1 vegan substitute for fish oils, as they can contain just as many fatty acids. Omega 3 acids are also said to enhance exercise performance. You will be able to exercise for longer hours.

Nutrients

Walnuts are rich in multiple nutrients, including B vitamins and zinc—these aid in keeping the immune system healthy. You will fall sick less often and be able to perform better.

Almonds

Almonds are the second-best nuts to add to your diet. They are just as nutritious as walnuts, if not more.

Here is what makes almonds good for your body.

Calcium

Almonds contain a high dose of calcium required to maintain strong bones. Just by nibbling on a few almonds, you can increase the calcium content in your bones and prevent them from drawing from your bloodstream.

Fiber

The fiber content in almonds is extremely high, making them ideal for athletes. The body does not digest fiber and tricks it into working hard to digest it.

This causes the body to up its metabolism and assists with improving digestion.

Protein

Almonds have a fair amount of proteins that can contribute to your daily requirement. Munching on a few before and after your workout session can leave you energetic and help your muscles recover faster.

Magnesium

Magnesium is an important body component and is especially required by athletes to remain healthy. It helps enhance testosterone release and control cortisol, thereby enabling better performance.

Both walnuts and almonds can be added to smoothies or toasted and sprinkled over salads

Sweet potatoes

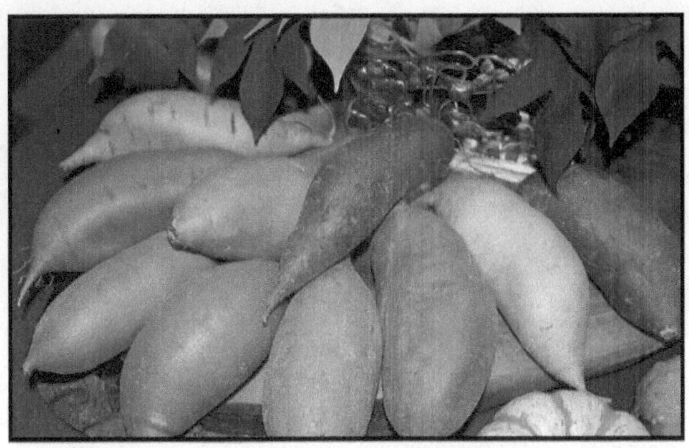

The next vegan superfood to add to your diet is sweet potatoes. Here is why you should make it a big part of your daily diet.

Energy

Sweet potatoes provide you with truckloads of energy. Consuming sweet potatoes, regardless of your sport, will surely experience a marked difference in energy levels. The energy will be consistent and last throughout the day.

Vitamin A

Sweet potatoes are loaded with vitamin A and can meet 100% of your daily requirement. Vitamin A is an essential antioxidant needed to boost your immune system. It checks infections and keeps you healthy from the inside out.

Inflammation

Sweet potatoes control inflammation to a large extent. Athletes run the risk of suffering from muscle inflammation. The best way to deal with this is by consuming sweet potatoes. Not only do they control inflammation, but they also help in reducing non-contact injuries.

Glycemic index

High glycemic foods spike up blood sugar levels in your body. Although this might seem ideal for an athlete, avoiding such foods as much as possible is essential as it can lead to the development of type 2 diabetes. Sweet potatoes happen to curb the release of sugars and control insulin levels in the bloodstream.

Complex carbs

Sweet potatoes consist of complex carbs that the body does not dig easily digest. This makes it an excellent food to consume post-workout, as the body will continue to burn fat. It also helps to add back some of the lost energy, so you have enough left to do the remaining chores.

Magnesium and potassium

Sweet potatoes contain magnesium and potassium, which help control muscle spasms. They also help in controlling cramps and improve muscle function. Any injured muscles will recover faster, thereby enhancing your performance drive.

Seeds (Chia and Sesame Seeds)

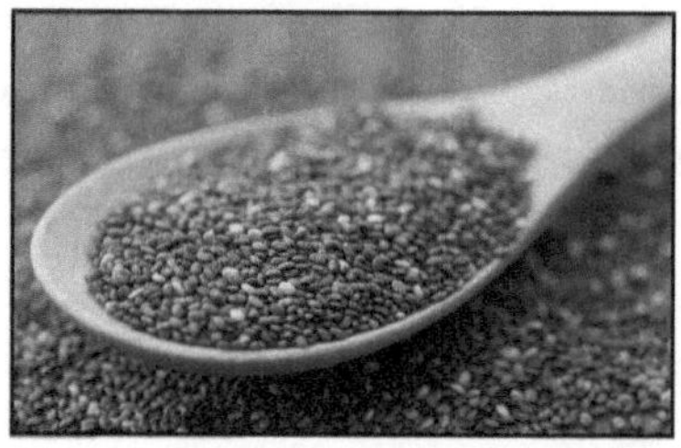

Chia seeds

Chia seeds are very nutritious and can provide athletes with sustained energy. They are favorites among runners and gym goers. Here are some of the health benefits.

Dehydration

Chia seeds can hold almost 30 times their weight in water and can, therefore, provide the body with consistent hydration. They are ideal for athletes and exercisers who work out in humid climates and require more hydration than others.

Joint aches

Rich in omega-3 fatty acids, Chia seeds help create a lubricating barrier between joints. This helps in reducing inflammation and facilitates movement. These oils also help in controlling hyperactivity and hypertension.

Weight loss

Since these seeds absorb far more water than their capacity, they can be consumed to feel fuller for longer. Again, a handful will do the job; you do not have to worry about feeling puckish between meals.

Recovery

The amino acids found in Chia seeds can help accelerate recovery time. It can decrease the time taken by your muscles to recover from soreness. They are, therefore, best eaten as soon as you step out of the gym or finish your exercise routine. A cup of Chia seeds can leave you with 10 grams of fiber.

Sesame seeds

Sesame seeds are the next best seeds to add to your diet. They might be tiny, but they are loaded with nutrition. Here are some of the health benefits provided by sesame seeds.

Calcium

Sesame seeds are a storehouse of calcium. Calcium is essential for all athletes as it can quickly deplete during workouts. Thirty grams of sesame seeds can provide the body with 350 grams of calcium. This makes for nearly 40% of the daily requirement.

Iron

Iron is required by the body to produce hemoglobin that transports oxygen to the different muscle tissues. Thirty grams of sesame seeds can provide you with 5 grams of iron, which happens to be 60% of the daily requirement for men.

Zinc

Studies show athletes and bodybuilders have a high risk of developing zinc deficiency. This can lead to fatigue, reduced endurance, and brain fog. Sesame seeds, rich in zinc content, can solve this problem once and for all. As a result, you will feel energetic and experience enhanced performance.

As you can see, chewing on a few chia and sesame seeds daily can help you enhance your athletic performance.

Banana

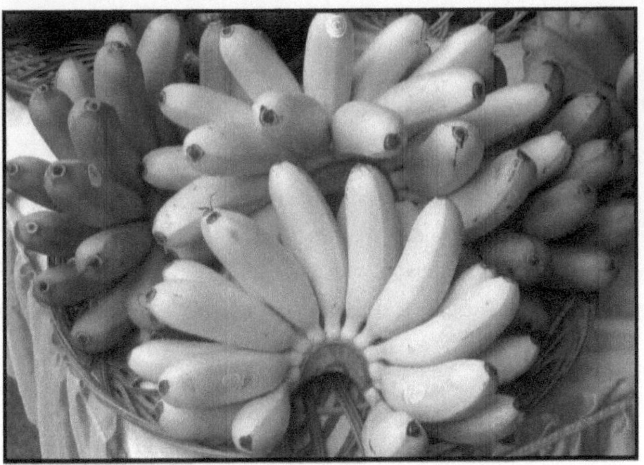

Rounding up the list of superfoods is the humble banana. Bananas are an athlete's ideal food, loaded with vital nutrients. They are as follows.

Potassium

Bananas are rich in potassium content. A banana has 450 mg of potassium, 14% of your daily requirement. Potassium helps in controlling blood sugar levels and can enhance heart function. Potassium can protect your heart by curbing high blood pressure. Athletes tend to feel dehydrated quite often. The best solution is to consume a banana, as it acts as

An electrolyte that balances body fluids. Potassium can also significantly reduce the occurrence of muscle cramps and contribute towards the development of stronger, leaner muscles.

Carbohydrates

A banana can contain 30 grams of carbohydrates, making it ideal for athletes. Consuming half a banana before a workout session will ensure that you have enough energy to last you through the day. You can follow up your workout with another half to regain lost energy. As per experiments conducted on gymnasts, bananas helped in improving their reflexes. Those who consumed a banana before their balance beam routines were able to stave off falls.

Vitamin C

A banana can give you 15% of your daily vitamin C requirement. Vitamin C is essential for strengthening muscles, ligaments, and tendons. It is also responsible for increasing immunity and providing fast relief from wounds- acquired while working out. It is also responsible for synthesizing the adrenaline required for daily exercise routines.

Bananas are readily available and relatively cheap. You can consume half a large banana before your workout and one after.

Superfoods are great for your body because of their nutritional content. It will do wonders for your health and energy. Not just that, but it will also speed up your workout recovery time! At the same time, you can strengthen your mind and build lean muscle. When working out, endurance, strength, and recovery are the most critical parts of the puzzle. I hope you develop the body of your dream and excel in your sport.

Vegan Recipes

New-To-You Food Guide

Cheese

Dairy-free cheeses are often made from nuts, soy, or tapioca. Nutritional yeast (see below) also adds a cheesy flavor to foods. Brands: Daiya, Parma, Teese, Tofutti, Treeline, Vegan Gourmet

Condiments

Condiments, including butter, mayo, and sour cream, are available in veg-friendly forms. Brands: Earth Balance, Just Mayo, Nayonaise, Tofutti, Vegan Gourmet, Vegenaise

Milk, Yogurt, and Ice Cream

Dairy-free products are made from almonds, coconut, flax, hemp, oats, rice, and soy. All are free of cholesterol. Brands: Almond Breeze, Coconut Bliss, Pacific, Silk, So Delicious, Tempt, Tofutti, Whole Soy

Nutritional Yeast

This flaky, inactive yeast has a cheesy flavor. Try substituting for parmesan on top of pasta, pizza, or any other food you'd like to add a cheesy taste. Fortified versions contain B vitamins, B12, and other essential minerals. Brands: Bragg, Red Star.

Seitan

Made from wheat gluten, seitan is packed with protein and offers a meaty texture when cooked. Brands: Upton's Naturals, West Soy

Tahini

A calcium-rich, creamy sesame seed paste often used in Middle Eastern cuisine.

Tempeh

Tempeh is a firm, fermented soybean product. It has a nutty flavor and can replace meat in a recipe. Brands: Lightlife, Tofurky

Tofu

Made from soybeans, tofu is popular in vegetarian recipes because it is high in protein and calcium and easily absorbs flavors. It comes in a white block that can be fried, sautéed, steamed, or used in smoothies. Check recipes to see whether you should use a firm or silken variety.

TVP/Vegan Crumbles

Textured Vegetable Protein (TVP) is a dried protein that must be soaked in liquid before adding to a recipe. Vegan crumbles can be used straight from the package. Both add a meaty texture to stew, chili, and pasta sauce. Brands: Beyond Meat, Bob's Red Mill, Gimme Lean.

Carrot Muffins

Makes 1 dozen

- 1 cup whole-wheat flour
- 1 cup oats or wheat bran
- 1 tablespoon cornstarch
- 2 teaspoons baking powder
- 1 teaspoon allspice
- ½ teaspoon ground cinnamon
- ½ teaspoon salt
- 1 cup raw carrots, grated
- 1 cup water
- $^1/_3$ cup sugar or maple syrup
- ¼ cup mild-flavored oil or vegan butter melted

Preheat the oven to 375

Combine flour, oats or bran, cornstarch, baking powder, allspice, cinnamon, and salt in a large mixing bowl. Toss in the grated carrots. Add the water, sugar or maple syrup, and oil or butter, and mix gently.

- Spoon the batter into a lightly oiled or lined muffin pan so each tin is about two-thirds full. Bake for 25-30 minutes or until an inserted toothpick comes out clean. Allow to cool in the pan for 5 minutes before transferring to a baking rack.

Pancakes

Serves 4

- 1 ½ cups all-purpose flour
- 1 tablespoon baking powder
- 1 tablespoon sugar

¼ teaspoon salt

- 2 ½ cups dairy-free milk
- 2 tablespoons vegetable oil

1. Heat a non-stick skillet over medium heat until a drop of water gently sizzles and pops.
2. Mix the dry ingredients in a large bowl. Whisk in the wet ingredients, being careful not to over-mix. If there are lumps, allow the batter to sit for a minute to break down.
3. Fill a quarter cup and pour batter onto the skillet. Cook over medium heat. Flip when the edges begin to dry and bubbles on the top start to pop.
4. Cook for another 1-2 minutes and serve with vegan butter, maple syrup, agave syrup, or fresh fruit.

Tofu French Toast

Makes 6-8 pieces

- 8 ounces of silken tofu
- ½ cup dairy-free milk
- 1 teaspoon agave or maple syrup
- ½ teaspoon cinnamon
- 1 ripe banana
- Vegan butter or mild-flavored oil for cooking
- 6-8 slices of bread
-

Heat a non-stick pan over medium heat.

- In a blender or food processor, blend the tofu, dairy-free milk, syrup, cinnamon, and banana until smooth. If too thick add a few tablespoons of extra dairy-free milk or water. Pour the coating mixture into a shallow dish and dip the bread into the mixture, completely coating both sides.
- Melt a teaspoon of oil or vegan butter on the hot skillet, and then add your soaked bread.
- Cook for 2-3 minutes and flip to cook the other side once the edges begin to turn golden brown. Repeat with remaining bread.
- Serve with fresh fruit, powdered sugar, or maple syrup.

Savory Breakfast Sandwiches

Makes 4 sandwiches

- ¼ cup apple cider vinegar
- 2 tablespoons soy sauce
- ¼ cup olive oil
- 1 teaspoon black pepper, divided
- 1 (14-ounce) package of firm tofu, drained and cut crosswise into 8 slices
- 1 large onion, chopped
- 3 cloves garlic, chopped
- 8 ounces button mushrooms, sliced
- 1 medium tomato, chopped
- 2 cups baby spinach leaves
- ¼ teaspoon dried thyme
- ½ teaspoon salt
- Vegan butter (optional)
- 4 English muffins, toasted

In a shallow baking dish, mix the vinegar, soy sauce, olive oil, and ½ teaspoon of black pepper with a whisk. Place tofu slices in a single layer in the dish, then turn over to coat on all sides. Allow tofu to marinate for 20 minutes, turning occasionally.

Place the baking dish in the oven for 20 minutes. Flip tofu slices over and continue to bake for an additional 10-20 minutes until crispy and most of the liquid has been absorbed.

1. Meanwhile, spray a large skillet with oil or cooking spray. Sauté onion and garlic over medium-high heat until the onion begins to soften. Add mushrooms and continue cooking until they begin to brown. Add tomato, spinach, thyme, salt, and remaining black pepper. Cook and stir until spinach is wilted and any liquid has evaporated, turning the heat to medium-low if the vegetables are browning too quickly. Adjust seasoning.
2. To assemble sandwiches, spread vegan butter on English muffins if using. Then add 2 tablespoons of the cooked vegetables to the bottom half of each muffin. Top with 2 slices of tofu and evenly distribute the remaining vegetables on top of the tofu slices on all 4 sandwiches. Cover with the other muffin halves and press down to help keep vegetables from spilling out.

Barbecue Seitan Sandwiches

Serves 4

- 1 tablespoon vegetable oil
- 1 small onion, chopped
- 1 package seitan strips or chunks cut into strips
- 1 cup vegan barbecue sauce

¼ cup water

- Hot sauce (optional)
- 4 hamburger buns

- Suggested toppings: lettuce, tomato, green pepper, coleslaw, red onions

1. Heat the vegetable oil in a large pan over medium heat. Add the onion and sauté for 5-8 minutes, or until the onion is very soft. Add seitan, and cook until lightly browned, stirring often.
2. Add the barbecue sauce and water and cook, stirring every 5 minutes, until the sauce has thickened and been absorbed by the seitan. Add hot sauce to taste if using.
3. Toast the inside of the buns to prevent them from getting soggy, then spoon the seitan mixture onto the rolls and garnish. Serve hot.

Black Bean Soup

Serves 6-8

- 2 tablespoons olive oil
- 1 onion, chopped
- 3 cloves garlic, minced
- 1 green bell pepper, chopped
- 1 can diced tomatoes
- 2 tablespoons white or apple cider vinegar
- 1 teaspoon ground cumin
- ¼ cup fresh parsley

  1 teaspoon ground coriander

- 1 teaspoon smoked paprika
- 3-4 bay leaves
- Salt and pepper to taste
- 6 cups black beans, cooked
- 2 cups vegetable broth

In a large stockpot over medium-high heat, sauté the onion, garlic, and bell pepper in the olive oil until the onion begins to soften, about 5 minutes.

Add the tomato, vinegar, cumin, coriander, paprika, bay leaves, salt, and pepper, and cook for another 5 minutes.

Add the beans and broth and reduce to a simmer. Cook for about 15 minutes, covered.

Remove bay leaves.

Serve garnished with parsley

Serves 8

Chili

1 cup dry TVP or 1 package vegan crumbles (optional)

1 tablespoon vegetable oil

1 large onion, coarsely chopped

1 28-ounce can of diced tomatoes

1 small can of tomato paste

1 jalapeño pepper, minced (optional)

3 tablespoons chili powder (or more to taste)

½ teaspoon ground cumin

2 teaspoons garlic powder

2 teaspoons Italian seasoning

1 teaspoon salt

Black pepper to taste

½ cup vegetable broth

2 carrots, chopped

1 bell pepper, chopped

2 15-ounce cans of beans drained and rinsed (kidney, black, pinto, etc.), add a   third can of beans if not using vegan crumbles or TVP

1 cup frozen corn

1 med zucchini, chopped

If using TVP, start by heating a few teaspoons of vegetable oil in a large skillet. Add the TVP and toast over medium-high heat, stirring constantly for about 3 minutes. Toasting the TVP will give the texture a bit more of a bite and keep it from getting soggy. Bring 1 cup of water or vegetable broth to a boil and pour over the TVP. Set aside.

4. In a large stockpot, heat 1 tablespoon of vegetable oil over medium heat. Add the onion and cook for about 2 minutes. Next add the diced tomatoes, tomato paste, jalapeño (if using), chili powder, ground cumin, garlic

powder, Italian seasoning, salt, and pepper, and allow to cook for about 5 minutes.

5. Add the broth, soaked TVP or vegan crumbles (if using), carrots, and bell pepper. Cover and turn down the heat. Simmer for 30 minutes.
6. Add the beans, corn, and zucchini and simmer uncovered for an additional 30 minutes.
7. Adjust seasoning to taste and serve with rice or pasta and top with vegan sour cream, if desired.

Egg-Free Salad Sandwiches

Makes 4 sandwiches

- 1 12-ounce package of extra firm tofu
- ½ cup vegan mayonnaise
- 2 teaspoons mustard
- 1 teaspoon lemon juice or apple cider vinegar
- 1 teaspoon garlic powder
- ¼ teaspoon ground cumin
- 1 celery stalk, diced
- 1 small pickle, diced
- 2 green onions, diced
- Salt and pepper to taste
- ¼ teaspoon Black Salt (kala namak) (optional)
- Bread, tomato, lettuce, or other desired sandwich fixings
-

Wrap the tofu in a paper towel, then a clean dish towel. Press by leaving between two heavy pots for about 10 minutes. Replace the soaked dish towel with another dry towel and press for another 5 minutes. Or use a tofu press. Chop up the tofu into nonuniform chunks or cubes.

Toss tofu in a bowl with vegan mayonnaise, mustard, lemon juice or vinegar, garlic powder, and cumin. Stir in the celery, pickle, and onions. Season with salt, pepper, and black salt if using. Use less salt if also using black salt, which adds a great eggy flavor.
Toast bread before assembling your sandwiches and serve with your favorite fixings.

Cooking without Eggs, vegan substitutes

Use any of these
tips to replace
one egg when
making cakes,
muffins,
pancakes, and
bread.

- 2 tablespoons cornstarch med
with 1 tablespoon water

- Half a banana, mashed

- ¼ cup silken tofu

- 1 tablespoon flax meal mixed
with 1 tablespoon water

- ¼ cup applesauce + ½ teaspoon
baking powder

- Ener-G Egg Replacer, follow
directions on box

- 1 teaspoon The Vegg Baking Mix,
mix with ¼ cup water

Lasagna

Serves 6

- 1 14-ounce package of extra firm tofu
- 1 tablespoon lemon juice or white vinegar
- 1 teaspoon salt
- 1 teaspoon garlic powder
- 1 teaspoon Italian seasoning
- ¼ teaspoon ground nutmeg
- 1 package vegan crumbles or 2 cups TVP
- 2 cups vegetable broth, if using TVP
- 1 tablespoon olive oil
- 6 cups red marinara sauce
- 1 12-ounce package of lasagna noodles
- 8 ounces of raw spinach
- ½ cup vegan mozzarella shreds

1. Preheat the oven to 375°F.

To create tofu ricotta, drain and mash the tofu in a mixing bowl. Add the lemon juice, salt, garlic powder, Italian seasoning, and nutmeg. Set aside.

2. If using vegan crumbles, break them up in a small frying pan with a tablespoon of olive oil. Fry for about 5 minutes, stirring occasionally. Once it starts to turn golden and crispy, remove it from the heat. If using TVP, soak it in the 2 cups of boiling broth.
3. Spread a thin layer of marinara sauce on the bottom of a 9 x 13-inch pan.
4. Prepare the dry noodles by spreading the tofu ricotta evenly on each piece. Place 1 layer of noodles on the bottom of the pan. Place a layer of spinach leaves on top of the noodles, followed by half of the vegan crumbles or TVP.
5. Then pour 1 cup of marinara sauce, making sure it is evenly distributed over the whole pan. Repeat with the second half of your ingredients. Top with a final layer of noodles, the last cup of marinara sauce, and a half cup of vegan cheese.
6. Cover with foil and bake for 35-45 minutes, until the sauce is bubbling. Uncover and bake for an additional 5 minutes. Allow to cool and set for at least 15 minutes before serving.

"unmeat Meatloaf"

Serves 4-6

- 1-pound vegan crumbles
- ½ cup soft bread crumbs
- ¼ cup dairy-free milk
- 1 small onion, minced
- 3 cloves garlic, minced
- ¼ cup ketchup or tomato paste
- 1 tablespoon soy sauce
- 1 tablespoon mustard

- 1 teaspoon horseradish
- 1 teaspoon salt

Glaze

- ¼ cup ketchup or tomato paste
- 1 tablespoon mustard
- 1 tablespoon apple cider vinegar
- 1 tablespoon molasses

2. Preheat oven to 350°F.
3. Combine all of the meatloaf ingredients in a large bowl and mix thoroughly. Line a bread loaf pan with parchment paper and press the loaf ingredients into it.
4. Whisk together the glaze ingredients and spread evenly across the top of the loaf.
5. Cover the pan with foil and bake for 50 minutes. Uncover and bake for another 10 minute

Roasted Lemon Garlic "unchicken Chicken"

Serves 4

- 8 small red potatoes, quartered
- ¼ cup olive oil
- 2 lemons, 1 cut into thin slices or wedges, and 1 juiced

-8 cloves garlic, minced

1 teaspoon salt
- ½ teaspoon black pepper
- ¾ pound green beans trimmed
- 1 package of vegan chicken cutlets

3 sprigs of fresh rosemary, de-stemmed

1. Preheat oven to 400°F. Place the potatoes on a large baking sheet and toss them with a tablespoon of olive oil. Sprinkle with some salt and pepper. Roast for about 15 minutes while preparing the rest of the ingredients. This step will form a nice skin on the potatoes.
2. Coat a large baking dish or cast-iron skillet with 1 tablespoon of olive oil. Arrange the lemon slices and $^1/_3$ of the rosemary in a single layer on the bottom of the dish or skillet.
3. In a large bowl, combine the remaining olive oil and rosemary with the lemon juice, garlic, salt, and pepper; add the green beans and toss to coat. Using tongs, remove the green beans and arrange them on top of the lemon slices. Remove the potatoes from the oven and arrange them along the edge of the dish or skillet on top of the green beans.
4. Place the vegan chicken in the same bowl as the olive oil mixture and coat thoroughly. Place the chicken onto the skillet and pour any of the remaining olive oil mixtures over the top.
5. Roast in the oven for 20-30 minutes or until the green beans are tender, but still bright, and the chicken is golden brown around the edges. Place a piece of the roasted chicken on each serving plate and divide the green beans and potatoes equally. Top with the lemon slices and serve hot.

Egg-Free Potato Salad

Serves 6

- 2 pounds red potatoes, cut into large cubes
- $^1/_3$ cup vegan mayonnaise
- 2 tablespoons Dijon or brown mustard
- 1 tablespoon lemon juice
- 1 ½ teaspoons salt
- 1 teaspoon black pepper
- 1 cup celery, diced (optional)
- ¼ cup red onion, chopped (optional)
- ¼ cup parsley or chives, finely chopped

Bring a large pot of water to a rolling boil, then carefully add the chopped potatoes. Cook for about 10 minutes or until potatoes are soft enough to be pierced with a fork, but not at all mushy. Drain and rinse in cold water. Set aside to cool completely.

1. Separately, combine the mayonnaise, mustard, lemon juice, salt, and pepper in a small bowl and mix well to combine.
2. When the potatoes are fully cooled, place them in a large bowl with the celery, onion, and parsley or chives. Mix gently to combine. Add the mayonnaise mixture and toss to coat. Cover and chill for at least 2 hours. Adjust seasoning before serving.

Creamy Mac & Cheese

Serves 2-4

- ½ pound pasta
- 1 tablespoon mustard
- 1 tablespoon lemon juice or apple cider vinegar
- 1 tablespoon soy sauce
- 1 tablespoon peanut butter or tahini

1 teaspoon garlic powder

- ½ teaspoon paprika
- 1 cup nutritional yeast
- 2 cups of dairy-free milk
- 1-2 teaspoons salt

- ½ cup vegan cheese shreds (optional)

1. Cook the pasta until al dente (cooked through, but still slightly firm). After draining the pasta, use the hot stockpot to cook your sauce.
2. Combine the mustard, lemon juice, soy sauce, and peanut butter (or tahini) in the stockpot over low heat. Add the garlic powder, paprika, and nutritional yeast, whisking to combine. Slowly add the dairy-free milk, a little at a time, until it reaches your desired thickness. Add salt and adjust to taste.
3. Add the vegan cheese if desired and cook until the cheese is completely melted. Turn off the heat and add the pasta, tossing to coat all the noodles.

Stuffing

- Serves 6-8

- 2 tablespoons vegetable oil, divided
- ½ small onion, diced
- 2 celery stalks, chopped
- 4 cups bread cubes, toasted
- 1 cup vegetable broth

- 2 Fuji, gala, or pink lady apples, cored and chopped $^1/_3$ cup raisins
- ¼ cup dried cranberries
- 1 teaspoon basil
- 1 teaspoon garlic powder
- 1 teaspoon oregano
- Salt and pepper, to taste

1. Preheat the oven to 350°F.

In a large skillet, heat 1 tablespoon of the oil. Sauté the onion and celery until tender, about 5- 7 minutes.

1. Use the remaining oil to grease a medium casserole dish and pour the sautéed vegetables into the dish.

2. Add all the remaining ingredients and toss well, making sure all of the bread cubes are soaked in the vegetable broth. Bake for 45 minutes.

Chocolate Chip Cookies

Makes 25-30 cookies

- 1 cup vegan butter, softened
- ½ cup white sugar
- ½ cup brown sugar
- ¼ cup dairy-free milk
- 1 teaspoon vanilla

- 2 ¼ cups flour
- ½ teaspoon salt
- 1 teaspoon baking soda
- 12 ounces of dairy-free chocolate chips

1. Preheat oven to 350°F.

2. In a large bowl, mix the butter, white sugar, and brown sugar until light and fluffy. Slowly stir in the dairy-free milk and then add the vanilla to make a creamy mixture.

3. In a separate bowl, combine the flour, salt, and baking soda. Add this dry mixture to the liquid mixture and stir well. Fold in the chocolate chips.

4. Drop small spoonfuls of the batter onto non-stick cookie sheets and bake for 8-10 minutes.

Brownies

Makes 20 brownies

- 2 cups flour
- 2 cups sugar

- ½ cup cocoa powder
- 1 teaspoon baking powder
- ½ teaspoon salt
- 1 cup vegetable oil (½ cup can be substituted with apple sauce for a more cake-like brownie) 1 cup water
- 1 teaspoon vanilla
- 1 cup dairy-free chocolate chips (optional)
- ½ cup chopped walnuts (optional)

1. Preheat oven to 350°F and grease a 9 x 13-inch baking pan.
2. Combine dry ingredients in a mixing bowl. Whisk together the wet ingredients and fold them into the dry ingredients. If desired, add half the chocolate chips and chopped walnuts to the mix. Pour mixture into the prepared pan and sprinkle with remaining chocolate chips and walnuts, if using.
3. For fudge-like brownies, bake for 20-25 minutes. For cake-like brownies, bake 25-30 minutes. Let the brownies cool slightly before serving.

Serves 6-8

- 16 to 24 ounces of silken tofu
- 2 cups pumpkin purée
- ¾ cup maple or agave syrup

- ¾ cup evaporated cane sugar
- ¼ cup cornstarch
- 1 teaspoon vanilla extract

cloves
- 1 9-inch unbaked pie shell

- 2 teaspoons ground cinnamon
- 1 teaspoon ground ginger
- ½ teaspoon ground nutmeg
- ½ teaspoon salt
- ¼ teaspoon ground

Preheat the oven to 400°F.

a. Combine the filling ingredients in a blender or food processor and blend until completely smooth. Pour the mixture into the pie shell.
b. Bake for 30 minutes, then turn down the oven temperature to 350°F. Bake for another 30-45 minutes or until the center of the pie appears set.
c.

Remove from oven and allow to cool completely. Chill for at least 2 hours to allow the pie to firm up even more.

Serves 2-4

Cake

- ¼ cup vegetable oil
- 1 tablespoon apple cider vinegar
- 2 teaspoons vanilla extract
- 1 ¼ cup dairy-free milk
- 2 cups all-purpose flour
- ¾ cup sugar
- 1 ½ teaspoons baking powder
- ½ teaspoon baking soda
- ½ teaspoon salt

Cake

1. Preheat oven to 350°F. Prepare a cupcake tin by placing baking liners into each of the cups.
2. In a small bowl, slowly mix the oil, vinegar, and vanilla into the dairy-free milk, allowing it to curdle. In a large bowl, sift together the flour, sugar, baking powder, baking soda, and salt.
3. Pour the liquid mixture over the flour mixture and stir gently, being very careful not to over-mix. Once combined, spoon the batter into each of the lined cupcake cups, filling each about two-thirds of the way full.
4. Bake for 20-25 minutes or until a toothpick inserted into the center of a cake comes out clean. Remove from oven and allow to cool for a few minutes in the tray. Once cool enough to touch, remove from the tray and cool the rest of the way on a cookie rack.

Buttercream Frosting

- 1 cup vegan butter
- 3-4 cups powdered sugar
- 1 teaspoon vanilla extract
- ¼ teaspoon salt
- 3-4 tablespoons of dairy-free milk
-

Buttercream Frosting

2. While the cupcakes are cooling, prepare the buttercream. Start by whipping the vegan butter with an electric mixer or by hand until slightly soft and smooth. Add the powdered sugar, 1 cup at a time. Add the full 4 cups for a sweeter and stiffer frosting.
3. Mix in the vanilla, salt, and a little bit of dairy-free milk until your desired consistency is reached. Spread or pipe the frosting onto the completely cooled cupcakes in whatever fashion you like and enjoy.

AVOCADO BRAIN-BOOSTER SMOOTHIE

½ frozen banana
¼ avocado
¼ cup frozen blueberries

1 handful spinach

1 cup almond milk

1 tsp ground flax seed

1 scoop vegan protein powder (optional)

Add all ingredients to the blender, and blend until smooth.

STRAWBERRY COCONUT SMOOTHIE

½ cup coconut milk

½ cup water

½ banana (frozen),

1 cup frozen strawberries

1 Tbsp unsweetened shredded coconut

¼ tsp vanilla extract

1/8 tsp cinnamon

1 scoop vegan protein powder (optional)

ADD ALL INGREDIENTS TO THE BLENDER,
AND BLEND UNTIL SMOOTH.

Apple Carrot

2 apples, cored
4 carrots, ends trimmed
¼ cucumber
1-inch fresh ginger peeled

Cut apple.
Put all ingredients into blender *carrots, apples, cucumber, and ginger.*

serve immediately.

Turnip and Carrots

The turnip is a much-underrated vegetable. With these two vegetables, you're getting plenty of vitamins A and C.

Ingredients:

3 carrots

½ turnip

1 cup strawberries.

Directions:

Peel the turnip before processing the ingredients in the juicer.

Sweet Spinach

This is perfect if you don't like spinach, because you'll barely taste it. You'll just enjoy the benefits

Ingredients:

1 apple

1 cup spinach

1 orange

Bunch of parsley

Directions:

Process the ingredients in the juicer.

Pineapple Delight

The fruit helps sweeten the Swiss chard

Ingredients:

1 apple

1 cup strawberries

8 chard leaves

1 cup pineapple

Handful of parsley

Directions:

Process all ingredients in the juicer.

Merry Berry Peach

Asparagus is a mild vegetable, so it blends easily with fruit and berries. You don't have to, but it's probably better to remove the tough stems from the asparagus before juicing.

Ingredients:

4 asparagus

1 pitted peach

1 cup blueberries

1 cup spinach

Directions:

Trim the asparagus and process the fruits and vegetables through the juicer.

Raspberry Surprise

Ingredients:

1 cup raspberries

1 cup spinach

½ cup pineapple

3 carrots

Directions:

Feed all ingredients into your juicer.

Rise and Shine Juice

Ingredients:

2 apples

2 carrots

2 oranges

Directions:

Slice but don't peel the apples. Peel the oranges.

Process all ingredients through the juicer.

Green Juice

This is a great juice anytime, but it's an especially good detox when you've overdone the fun, such as on vacations or during the holidays.

Ingredients:

2 apples

1 peach

1 cucumber

1 bunch of collard greens

Directions:

Cut up the fruit, peach, cucumber, and greens and process in the juicer.

<u>Watermelon Smoothie</u>

Ingredients:

3 cups chunked watermelon

3 cups ice

1 banana

1 cup chunked cantaloupe

½ cup apple juice

2 tbsp. agave nectar

Directions:

Combine all ingredients in a blender. Blend until smooth, serve immediately.

Carrot and Orange Juice

Ingredients:

1 lb. peeled and sliced carrots

3 peeled oranges

1 cup pineapple

½-inch piece of ginger

Bunch of parsley

Directions:

Process the carrots, pineapple, and oranges in the juicer first, then add the ginger and parsley

VEGAN EATING ON A BUDGET

Whether you're a student, raising a family on a tight budget, or just saving for the future, choosing vegan foods doesn't mean breaking the bank. There are plenty of nutritious vegan options that are as economical as they are tasty. Here are some meal ideas to help you discover how easy—and affordable—it is to transition to a more compassionate diet:

Breakfast

- Oatmeal with fruit or maple syrup
- Cereal with soy milk and sliced bananas
- Peanut butter or jam on toast or a bagel
- Smoothie of fresh or frozen fruit with soy milk

Lunch/Dinner

- Rice, beans, and vegetables on a platter or in a tortilla
- Pasta with marinara sauce and frozen veggies
- Baked sweet potato topped with salsa, baked beans, or veggie chili
- Lentil soup with veggies

Snacks

- Celery, apples, or carrots topped with peanut butter or hummus
- Popcorn seasoned with nutritional yeast or salt
- Make-your-own trail mix with nuts, raisins, and sunflower seeds

Thank you for purchasing

The Beginner Vegan Athlete

Carol Capper

ABOUT THE AUTHOR

Carol Capper has published multiple books on health and wellness with the beginner in mind. Carol holds multiple free weekly vegan classes on her website for those interested in going vegan.
www.onesourceconsulting.net
Carol lives in the Midwest with her husband and three fur babies.